THE DOCTOR'S GUIDE TO

DIABETES

AND YOUR CHILD

THE DOCTOR'S GUIDE TO
DIABETES
AND YOUR CHILD

New Therapies for
Type 1 and Type 2

ALLAN E. SOSIN, M.D.
with Sheila Sobell

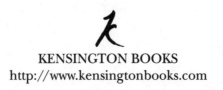

KENSINGTON BOOKS
http://www.kensingtonbooks.com

The recommendations made in this book should be followed only under the direction of a physician. This book is not intended to replace or contradict professional guidance. If you or your child is undergoing medical treatment, consult with your physician before making any changes in the medical regimen.

The names and identities of patients have been changed to protect their privacy. The author and publisher are not responsible in any way for products or services mentioned in this book.

KENSINGTON BOOKS are published by

Kensington Publishing Corp.
850 Third Avenue
New York, NY 10022

All Kensington titles, imprints and distributed lines are available at special quantity discounts for bulk purchases for sales promotion, premiums, fund raising, educational or institutional use.

Special book excerpts or customized printings can also be created to fit specific needs. For details, write or phone the office of the Kensington Special Sales Manager: Kensington Publishing Corp., 850 Third Avenue, New York, NY, Attn. Special Sales Department. Phone: 1-800-221-2647.

Kensington and the K logo Reg. U.S. Pat. & TM Off.

ISBN 1-57566-576-X

First Kensington Trade Paperback Printing: November, 2000
10 9 8 7 6 5 4 3 2 1

Printed in the United States of America

To my wife, Susan and sons Nicholas, Jonathan, and Benjamin, without whom I would know nothing.

To Glenn Doman and his staff, who have demonstrated for half a century what marvels parents and children can create with good information.

To Julian Whitaker, who has worked to demystify medicine.

To Jeffrey Bland, who promotes the therapy of people as individuals.

To Paul Doolan, a great teacher at the right time.

And to Richard Nicholas Every, Sheila Sobell's husband, who makes life's magic possible.

ACKNOWLEDGMENTS

Diane Lara, clinical nutritionist, created all the recipes in this book. They were tested in her kitchen and in the Sosins' kitchen by assorted Sosins and guests.

Thanks to Susan Sosin for the benefit of her suggestions, support, and experience.

Thanks to Lee Heiman for his advice and encouragement, to Claire Gerus, to Peggy Dace and Kelley Griffin, and to Richard Ember.

CONTENTS

Foreword xi
Testimonial xiii
Introduction xvii

PART I: THE CHALLENGE OF DIABETES 1

Chapter 1: Getting the Facts Straight 3

The Faces of Diabetes 3
What Is Diabetes 6
Blood-Sugar Levels: What's Too High? What's Too Low? 7
What Insulin Does 9
Juvenile Diabetes (Type 1) 10
Possible Triggers of Type 1 Diabetes 11
Pancreatic Damage and the Onset of Diabetes 13
Insulin Administration 14
Outlook for Juvenile Diabetes 16
Adult-Onset (Type 2) Diabetes 18
Adult-Onset Diabetes Affects Children Too 19
Type 2 Diabetes in Children: An Emerging Epidemic 20
Diagnosing Type 2 Diabetes 21
The First Symptoms of Type 2 Diabetes 21
The Role of Genetics 22
Preventing Long-Term Complications 23
The Outlook for Type 2 Diabetes 28
The Drug Approach: Type 1 28
The Drug Approach: Type 2 29
Drug Dangers 30
Rezulin: A Cautionary Tale 32
The Challenge of Diabetes 34

Chapter 2: Diabetes Is a Family Affair 36

Gaining Control 38
How Fear Paralyzes Learning 38

Changing the Family Dynamic 40
Involving Your Child in Diabetes Management 41
Considering Home Schooling 42
Demystifying Diabetes Management 43

Chapter 3: The Great American Obesity Epidemic 46

Measuring Obesity 46
Insulin and Weight Gain 50
Genetics Not Always Destiny 52
The Energy Equation 53
Television and Obesity 54
Food in the Fast Lane 54
Obesity and Cancer 57
Aren't French Fries Vegetables? 59

Chapter 4: High-Risk Foods 61

The Trouble with Cow's Milk 61
America's Deadly High-Fat Diet 63
Dietary Fats and Diabetes 64
Terrible Trans-Fatty Acids 65
High-Protein Diet Problems 67
Processed Carbohydrates and Sugar: A Shortcut to Diabetes 69
Whole Grains and Vegetables to the Rescue 70
Enriched Flour: A Poor Choice 71
Sugar and Empty Calories 71
Sugars Added to Foods 73
Turning Kids into Sugar Junkies 75
Aspartame 76
Sweet Solutions 77
Dangers of Food Enhancers 79
MSG: The Unsavory Truth 80
The Business of Food 81

Chapter 5: A Safer Environment 83

Your Drinking Water 83
Buying Pesticide-Free 87

Are Genetically Engineered Foods Safe? 88
Protect Your Kids Against Environmental Toxins 90

PART II: GETTING WELL 93

Chapter 6: Food as Medicine 95

Weight Control 96
The Truth About Eggs 99
Taking the Initiative 101
Only One Healthy Anti-Diabetes Diet 102
Putting It All Together 103
Diet and Blood-Sugar Fluctuations 105
Exchange Lists—Why You Don't Need Them 106
Fiber Helps Control Blood Sugar 106
The Glycemic Index 108
Using the Glycemic Index 108
The Glycemic Index Is Not the Ten Commandments 111
Making the Index Work for You 112
Overcoming Dietary Misinformation 114
Managing Diabetes Takes Work 117

Chapter 7: Exercise and Supplements 119

Exercise May Be More Important Than Diet 119
Get Your Family Moving! 122
Exercise and Insulin 123
Get in the Exercise Habit Early 125
The Role of Supplements 126
Special Nutrients for Diabetic Children 127
Antioxidants 129
Magnesium 133
Chromium 134
Vanadium 135
B Vitamins 136
Gymnema Sylvestre 136
Essential Fatty Acids 137

Chapter 8: Parents and Children: Partners in Healing 141

Parents' Questions About Getting Well 145
Pharmaceutical Advances in Controlling Diabetes 146
Helping Kids to Make Wise Food Choices 147
Using Nutritional Supplements 148
Incorporating Exercise 148
Encourage Your Kids to Share Their Feelings 149
A Child's Health Crisis Can Draw the Family Closer 150
Developing Good Health Habits 151
28 Tips for Keeping Your Child Healthy 152

Chapter 9: The Nutritional Program   162

Helpful Hints 162
Breakfast Suggestions and Combinations 167
Lunches for School or at Home 174
Dinner Recipes 177
Dessert Recipes 186
Drinks 195

Appendix I: Proper Eating/Shopping Guide 197

Appendix II: Resources 201

Glossary 237
Selected References 249
For Further Reading 257
Index 259

Foreword

Dr. Allan Sosin, a close colleague of mine and former medical director of the Whitaker Wellness Institute, has written a book of vital importance to parents. The increasing incidence of diabetes, which experts predict will reach epidemic proportions in the next decade, is cause for great concern. It's very alarming that this condition, which used to be primarily associated with aging, is now affecting our children.

Never before have people eaten such high-calorie diets and been so sedentary. The resulting weight gain and obesity that now affect a majority of American adults have trickled down to our children. As a consequence, they—like us—are suffering from a multitude of health problems, including diabetes, weight problems, and nutritional deficiencies.

Dr. Sosin incisively addresses this cluster of conditions from two points of view: prevention and treatment. He offers a concise, easy-to-implement preventive program for the maintenance and enhancement of our children's health. Nowhere is prevention more important than in childhood, for health habits acquired in our youth tend to persist for life. In addition, propensities for later disease often have their start in our early years.

He also presents cutting-edge recommendations for the treatment of diabetes, weight problems, and nutritional deficiencies. And he goes beyond simply keeping blood-sugar levels under control to the actual prevention of complications of the eyes, kidneys, nerves, and cardiovascular system, which are so frequent in diabetics.

Both Dr. Sosin and I believe that treatment of diabetes must first and foremost be nutrition-based. The drumbeat that conventional medicine marches to—whatever the problem, prescribe a drug to fix it—is inappropriate and, in my opinion, unethical. Because so much solid research demonstrates the healing power of diet, exercise, and targeted nutritional supplements for this condition, these measures should be standard diabetes therapy for both children and adults.

This book's great strength is Dr. Sosin's ability to simplify what has traditionally been a very complicated disease to manage. Early in his career he learned how helping people achieve a sense of control over the management of their illness could transform them from victims to survivors with an optimistic attitude vital to achieving good health.

As a leader in the care of "impaired" children who would otherwise be relegated to custodial institutions, Dr. Sosin saw firsthand how application of very straightforward nutritional principles could transform the health of young people afflicted with grave illnesses like cerebral palsy, brain defects, and Down's syndrome.

With the publication of this book, Dr. Sosin brings the same thoughtful, caring style, insight, and commitment to the management of children with diabetes. *The Doctor's Guide to Diabetes and Your Child* offers an exciting challenge to the conventional approach to diabetes. As a society, we are long overdue for a shift from the current drug mentality to a more holistic approach to disease prevention and management. Allan Sosin strikes a thoughtful, well-researched blow at the outdated high-medication approach. Above all, he offers health and hope to our most precious resource—our children.

Julian M. Whitaker, M.D.
President and Founder
Whitaker Wellness Institute
Newport Beach, California

Testimonial

My son has Type 1 diabetes. Though he has always been very conscientious about monitoring his blood glucose levels, even with the best of care, problems can occur. Recently he had a stomach virus or food poisoning. He began to vomit after taking his insulin. This can be very dangerous for a diabetic. Because the illness did not resolve quickly, my son needed more information than he previously had about managing his diabetes. I knew this book was going to be published by Kensington, who had already published two of my books, so I called and asked for an early copy. What I found was a world of information for my son. This book contains nutritional and dietary information that individuals will probably not hear about from any other source. It is a must-read for anyone with Type 1 or Type 2 diabetes or for anyone who helps care for someone with diabetes.

Mary Ann Block, D.O.
Medical Director, the Block Center
Author, *No More Ritalin, No More Antibiotics*
and *Today I Will Not Die*

Introduction

How I got here

My odyssey through medicine is more than 30 years long. During that time, two objectives have remained consistent: to learn and to offer something of value. The path to learning, however, was not what I had anticipated.

What I learned in medical school was incomplete. We weren't taught the history of medicine or the evolution of medical thinking, nor did we learn about the effects on medicine of theology, superstition, and political and social upheavals. I didn't know that modern medicine was born from the victories of courageous scientists over useless medical conventions. Only in the last hundred years has medicine progressed to the point where it saves more people than it kills. Yet even now, the accepted "standard" of care includes outmoded and dangerous practices, and ignores newer and more humane measures.

I was initially interested in psychiatry, but came to see its methods as ineffective. After a couple of years in the Army, a year of travel in Europe, and a year of general medical practice, I began training in internal medicine. I developed a friendship with Dr. Paul Doolan, the head of my hospital. He was my first mentor, a perceptive, intense, and dedicated person with vast medical experience and a merciless way of cutting through pretense. He sensed my great need to succeed as a physician. He taught me to be attentive to all the details of a case, to have loyalty first to the patient and second to everything else. His lessons return to me now, lessons most of all in humility.

My wife, Susan, and I moved from Connecticut to New York City, where I studied nephrology, the diagnosis and treatment of kidney disease. I worked for Dr. Norman Deane, one of the pioneers of dialysis therapy for kidney failure. He liked to tell how dialysis had originally been maligned by leaders in the field of kidney disease, who claimed it could never work. They were wrong.

I was given the opportunity to set up programs for treating kidney failure using new techniques. I taught patients to perform continuous ambulatory peritoneal dialysis, a treatment that allowed them to manage their own therapy with a minimum of supervision. It was a wonderfully simple and effective method. People who had been miserable with other treatments were thriving. They were gaining control over their illness. As their teacher, I offered them the knowledge and skill to care for themselves. They changed from passive objects of therapy to individuals empowered to manage their own lives. I learned how important and satisfying it is to educate people to care for themselves.

What we have now in medicine is the opposite. We have the dreadful situation of patients dominated and alienated by cold and incomprehensible technology. Instead of understanding and trust, we have fear and anger. Adults, and especially children, require the knowledge to make them independent. This is the magic, the appeal, of "alternative medicine." It addresses people as thinking units capable of self-determination. It is right for people to want information more than they want authority. It makes sense to choose the approach that is least painful and damaging. Drugs and therapy are used in excess, often needlessly and with deleterious effect, when there are better methods of solving problems.

After we moved from New York to Philadelphia, my wife learned about an extraordinary place called The Institutes for the Achievement of Human Potential. Here, parents learned to improve their children physically, intellectually, and physiologically. I took a week off—not an easy thing to do in those days—to attend a "Better Baby" seminar. I was amazed. The Institutes offered new techniques for treating brain-injured children, and I saw children do things I did not think were possible at their age.

I saw children with brain defects, cerebral palsy, and Down's syndrome, performing at exceptional levels. These techniques worked so well that brain-injured children sometimes surpassed the expectations set for normal children.

In Philadelphia, I opened a practice in internal medicine. I also started working and learning at The Institutes, where I became assistant medical director for the next 14 years. I have remained emotionally and spiritually tied to that place and those people. It is immensely satisfying to know that such a place exists, that children otherwise relegated to custodial care can become productive and happy. Conversely, it is disturbing to observe the daily workings of our society and to see disease springing up everywhere. It is disturbing to see illness that can be prevented using simple measures of care, dedication to the welfare of children, and the application of straightforward nutritional principles.

The Institutes were founded by a physical therapist named Glenn Doman and a group of dedicated friends. Glenn has been the spiritual leader and main support for more than 40 years. Throughout that time, parents from many countries have brought their brain-injured children for help. These children have mild intellectual impairments or have been in a coma, or are blind, deaf, insensate, malnourished, convulsive, as rigid as boards or thoroughly limp, immobile, and constantly sick with one infection after another because their withered bodies can offer no resistance. After a complete evaluation, parents are offered intensive programs for the rehabilitation of their children. Success requires that these programs be followed throughout the day and sometimes through the night as well. The programs are difficult. They are followed for months or years. Sometimes parents are unable to continue.

But the results are amazing. With proper nutrition, vitamin and mineral supplements, detoxification from mind-numbing anti-convulsant drugs; with visual, auditory, and tactile stimulation; respiratory training, patterning (a method to teach the brain to initiate movement), balance training, crawling, creeping, running, gymnastics, music, reading and writing, these children survive. They awaken from coma, gain weight, stop having seizures, and no longer get sick. Runny noses, ear infections, pneumonia, and gastroenteritis no longer occur because their immune systems get stronger. Their heads and chests grow five times faster than before, and they grow taller at remarkable rates. This is called the catch-up phenomenon. The children begin to hear, to see, to feel, and to move for the first time. These changes are extraordinary to witness, and I saw them many times. Sometimes children graduate. They have attained normal function in the areas of speech, mobility, and manual dexterity.

Observing these miracles of human potential led me to wonder if these same techniques could improve the abilities of normal children. Could the standard of physical, intellectual, and psychological excellence be raised for all children? Were normal children receiving the best education, the best nutrition, the best exercise program?

There is certainly room for improvement in many areas. The impact of nutrition on health and performance is greatly ignored. Children who eat well will feel better, get sick less often, and accomplish more than children who do not. Children who are used to eating good foods are less likely to eat bad foods. I think they are also less likely to use drugs, alcohol, or cigarettes.

We can spare our children the diseases of modern life—obesity, inactivity, boredom, and mindless repetition. We can instill in them a desire to be healthy and to progress, to appreciate the wonder and variety of life. Our children's lives should not be detoured by mediocre television, fast foods, artificial tastes, passive interests, and passive behaviors. Normal children, too, have a right to succeed.

As my private practice grew, I looked for new therapies. I employed acupuncture with excellent results. I studied nutrition, went to conferences that explored lifestyle changes and their effect on health and disease. Eventually, my focus on illness became a focus on health. There is a big difference between the two.

I started patients on vitamins and minerals. I also treated them with chelation (a non-surgical treatment to rid the body of excess toxins, especially metals). I put together nutritional programs for them. My wife, Susan, became my nutritionist. I gave up coffee—and spent a weekend in bed with a headache. I gave up Coca-Cola, sugar, cheeseburgers, french fries and all other fast foods, candy bars, ice cream, bread, cakes, pies, cookies, fritos, meat, chicken, and gum. As a result, I lost 25 pounds and I felt fantastic.

The West Coast beckoned. The medical environment was changing. Managed care was gaining control of medicine in our area. I wanted to venture further into nutritional and alternative therapies, so I made contact with Dr. Julian Whitaker, a stalwart of wellness medicine who had spent time with Nathan Pritikin and had written books on the natural therapy of diabetes and heart disease. Dr. Whitaker also wrote the most popular medical newsletter in the country, with a monthly circulation of 500,000. His medical center in Newport Beach, California, held clinics where people came from around the country for one week. Whitaker offered them medical evaluations, nutritional instruction, lectures, and a "natural," non-drug and non-surgical approach to their problems. I went to work with him and became medical director of the center.

People who had been advised to submit to coronary angiography or bypass surgery, who had been made ill by prescription medications, and who had suffered other adverse effects of traditional therapies, came to our center for a second opinion. We were able to help them get off drugs, avoid surgery, and still resolve their problems. The education we provided empowered many of them to take control of their health for the first time. Patients who are dominated by dictatorial doctors do not fare well. We encouraged them to break free, to think for themselves, and to consider the least dangerous options first. Every patient is different and deserves respect for his or her own unique circumstances.

Why I wrote this book

The treatment of diabetes in this country is lacking in common sense. It is especially troubling to see children placed on rigorous programs of insulin and drug administration with only rudimentary instruction in proper diet and exercise. The use of nutritional supplementation is almost completely neglected. Parents are filled with bad stories, and they are terrified.

Beyond this, the trend toward obesity in this country has advanced undisturbed for the past thirty years. At present, over half of us are overweight and nearly a third of us are obese. Official warnings have had no effect. Obesity can lead to the most common type of diabetes in adults. Now our children are becoming increasingly overweight—over 25 percent at the present time—and are developing the adult form of diabetes at an alarming rate. The situation is getting worse because powerful commercial and societal forces are not being contested. The change we need is a lifestyle change. No drug will substitute for it.

This book provides parents with a program that will improve the treatment of their child's diabetes. It will help them and their child to better manage insulin-dependent, or Type 1, diabetes and to manage and prevent insulin-resistant, or Type 2, diabetes. By following this program, parents will improve the health of not just their diabetic child but their entire family as well.

I have treated hundreds of diabetic patients. Many were newly diagnosed and came looking for assistance in controlling their disease and preventing complications. Many had been diabetic for years, were experiencing side effects from medication or complications from the disease, and wanted to prevent further problems. Others had suffered severe complications, including blindness, kidney failure, heart failure, paralysis from stroke, or leg amputation. They wanted to improve their quality of life.

Only in the last decade has it been demonstrated that diabetic complications result from insufficient control of the blood sugar. The higher the blood sugar, the greater the damage to organs over time. It is important to realize that diabetes causes tissue damage over years, perhaps decades, and that any plan to prevent this damage must include a long-range program. This book provides such a program. It enables you to create a lifestyle that will ensure the most consistent regulation of blood-sugar levels as well as provide maximum protection for vulnerable organs.

Traditional medicine does not meet these needs. The current medical approach to diabetes is to find the right drug or combination of drugs and enforce compliance with a drug program. Thus, patients are being treated with a combination of various types of insulin, or insulin given by pump, or insulin given together with oral hypoglycemic agents, or various oral agents given together. I have seen patients who were prescribed Glynase plus Glucophage plus Rezulin, three different classes of drugs working at the same time to keep the blood sugar down. It is the drug therapy that receives precedence. The other factors in controlling diabetes—which are discussed in this book in detail—are ignored or provided only cursory attention.

Insulin causes hypoglycemia (abnormally low blood sugar). Oral hypoglycemics cause hypoglycemia plus a myriad of other side effects, some of which can be quite serious. A good example is Rezulin, a drug approved by the Food and Drug Administration (FDA) for use in the United States, despite being banned in England because of serious liver toxicity. Three years later, that drug has just been withdrawn from the market after causing dozens of deaths from liver failure. But not to fear, similar drugs are waiting in the wings to replace it, and we will see if they, too, cause liver problems.

I have seen many Type 2 diabetics who were able to entirely eliminate their need for drugs by making lifestyle changes and taking nutritional supplements to normalize the blood sugar. Ninety percent of diabetes is Type 2, and in many cases it is preventable or reversible without the need for medication. This book will show you how to do this through weight control, healthy eating practices, consistent exercise, and optimal nutritional supplementation.

These measures are not being taught by medical professionals. They know very little about nutrition and even less about the proper use of supplements. Meanwhile, many nutritionists are providing incorrect information to patients, permitting the use of undesirable foods that worsen diabetic control, raise blood pressure, and aggravate sugar cravings and obesity.

The most heartbreaking victims of this neglect have been children. That is why I wrote this book. I have seen child after child, brought in by worried or distraught parents, without a satisfactory treatment plan despite professional care. The parents were offered too little information, frightened sometimes to the point of panic by warnings of terrible diabetic complications awaiting their children.

Parents and their children need education, reassurance, and empowerment. They need to know how to manage Type 1 diabetes. They also need to know how to prevent and manage Type 2 diabetes, which becomes more common as people become more overweight, more sedentary, and more malnourished by processed foods that are depleted of nutrients. The same lifestyle measures recommended in this book for Type 1 diabetes will control and prevent Type 2 diabetes.

Parents like you who read this book should be reassured that your diabetic child can flourish and lead a long and happy life, that tragedy need not be waiting around the corner. You should realize that your other children, who may not be diabetic, are nevertheless at risk of serious future health problems unless they learn to follow a rational nutritional program. You should realize that you yourself are at risk of unhealthy diets, and that the changes you make for your children should also be for yourself.

I have always seen myself as a student. Yet the best student must also see himself as a teacher. As a teacher, one learns again the role of the student, learns what to ask and how to see. We are all ultimately both teacher and pupil. My patients have taught me more medicine than any professor or textbook. It is my pleasure to learn from them.

PART I

THE
CHALLENGE
OF
DIABETES

CHAPTER 1

Getting the Facts Straight

The Faces of Diabetes

Joanne

The news that 8-year-old Joanne had juvenile diabetes came as a major shock to her parents. On top of having three other demanding kids to raise, financial struggles, irritating incursions by the mother's parents on the family scene, and the father's obstructive and pig-headed boss, who made his job a living hell, they suddenly had to deal with a child's major illness. The ramifications were frightening.

They learned that Joanne was going to need insulin several times a day with injections in her thighs and abdomen, blood-sugar testing before breakfast, lunch, and dinner and before bed—and whenever else a problem was suspected. She was going to have at least four needle sticks in the fingers every day.

Joanne's first physician was an alarmist, type-A individual who managed to scare everyone. "Watch out for *low* blood sugars," he warned. "Joanne can have a seizure." Then he told them, "Watch out for *high* blood sugars also. Joanne can develop ketoacidosis, go into a coma, and die. Diabetics develop premature atherosclerosis, retinopathy, kidney disease, and neuropathy. If Joanne is not careful with blood-sugar control, she can go blind, require dialysis or a kidney transplant, lose her legs, or have heart failure or a stroke."

Joanne's parents were in a panic. Was the doctor's terrifying prognosis correct?

Kara

Kara had been skinny throughout her childhood, an active and happy tomboy who played baseball and soccer with the boys. She also loved dancing, especially tap dancing and ballet, and had received new red ballet shoes for her 12th birthday. She had a strong liking for Ritz crackers slathered with peanut butter and went to fast-food restaurants on weekends with her family. She attended the movies every week with her father, where he treated her to chocolate candy and popcorn.

On her 13th birthday, she fell out of a tree and broke her leg. She was admitted to the hospital, where she underwent surgery and was put in a cast for four months. The injury did not heal well enough for her to return to dancing. She missed her friends from the ballet class, and she became angry and frustrated. Her appetite for fast foods and snacks did not slacken. She replaced sports with television. By the time she was 17, she weighed 190 pounds.

There was a strong family history of Type 2, or adult-onset, diabetes on both her mother's and father's sides of the family. Her mother's sister had developed kidney failure and died after an unsuccessful renal transplantation.

One day Kara tripped and fell in the backyard, scraping her elbow. The elbow became red and raw and didn't heal. She went to a physician, who started her on antibiotics and, because he was suspicious, tested her urine. It revealed a high (256) concentration of sugar, more than a hundred points above normal. She also had high cholesterol of 280, an extremely high triglyceride level of 700, and a low level of HDL, or good cholesterol.

Kara was diagnosed as diabetic with Syndrome X. This is a combination of obesity, high cholesterol, and high triglycerides, frequently accompanied by high blood pressure and a tendency toward gout. People with Syndrome X are highly predisposed to complications of heart disease and stroke.

Kara's parents came to me with this question: "What do we do next?"

Larry

Larry's Type 1, or juvenile, diabetes was discovered when he was 3. He'd become lethargic, thirsty, and urinated a lot. His blood sugar was nine times normal (900) and ketones (compounds indicating an acid-base disturbance due to insufficient insulin) were present in his urine. He stayed in the hospital five days and was started on insulin.

When Larry was 5, his parents brought him to our clinic. He had been taking long- and short-acting insulin together before breakfast, short-acting insulin before dinner, and long-acting insulin before bed. His blood sugars were tested before breakfast, lunch, and dinner and at three in the morning. He often woke at one or two in the morning with hypoglycemic reactions, confused and flailing his arms.

The nutritionist at Larry's hospital had recommended a diet that included the following: Rice Krispies or Kix cereal with milk for breakfast, a similar dry cereal for a morning snack, four Diet Cokes a day, four glasses of 2-percent milk, graham or club crackers, ice cream, macaroni, bananas, rice, potatoes, melons, lunch meats, and his choice of American, provolone, or mozzarella cheese.

Larry's mother had been instructed to serve the food in measured portions in order to prevent the high glycemic-index foods (i.e., foods high in sugar) from elevating his blood sugar too much. But this diet was full of chemical additives and preservatives, trans fats, and other unhealthy ingredients. Worst of all, the diet was loaded with sugar and other simple carbohydrates that were guaranteed to produce rapid rises in blood sugar and demand large doses of insulin. In Larry's case, this led to an unfortunately all-too-common chain of events: the higher doses of insulin that were needed to bring his blood sugar down had lowered it too much. This was what caused his hypoglycemic reactions.

Larry's mother was confused. Couldn't she trust her child's dietician? What could Larry eat that would improve his condition, not worsen it?

Joanne, Kara, Larry, and their parents are typical of the diabetic children and worried families who come to my office. Parents are often overwhelmed by the complexity of this disease, baffled by their child's failure to thrive despite their best efforts, and depressed by what doctors tell them concerning the long-term implications of this life-threatening illness on young lives barely begun.

I spend a good part of these consultations listening to stories about how previously prescribed treatments have gone wrong and about the confusion, anxiety, and anger that diabetic children and their parents feel. I am enormously touched by these families and their wishes for their children to live full and satisfying lives despite diabetes. Understanding medical terms, learning how to test blood sugars, administer insulin, and master nutritional theory can be intellectually demanding and even daunting. This book will answer every parent's questions about diabetes and how to successfully manage it.

What Is Diabetes?

Diabetes mellitus is a disease characterized by excessive elevation of the blood-sugar level. There are two types of diabetes. Type 1 results from the failure of the pancreas to make sufficient amounts of insulin, the hormone that drives glucose (blood sugar) into the cells. It occurs mainly in children and young adults and must be treated with insulin.

Type 2 diabetes results from the resistance of the body's cells to the action of insulin, which usually is produced in normal amounts that increase in response to the body's resistance. This insulin resistance is often hereditary and is brought out by such factors as obesity, lack of exercise, improper food choices, and nutritional deficiencies. Controlling these factors will improve or even eliminate Type 2 diabetes. Controlling these factors will not eliminate Type 1 diabetes, but it will improve the control of blood sugar and thus help to prevent the complications of diabetes.

Keep in mind that both types of diabetes can cause the same complications, which are related to the degree of blood-sugar elevation and the way this can damage the body's tissues. These complications include cardiovascular disease, nerve damage, kidney disease, and eye disease.

Blood-Sugar Levels: What's Too High? What's Too Low?

The term you hear most often in connection with diabetes is blood sugar. What is blood sugar and why is maintaining it at specific levels so difficult yet so vital for a diabetic?

Blood sugar, or glucose, is the body's main source of energy. It is the fuel your cells use to produce energy. Glucose is obtained from carbohydrates in foods, which are absorbed through the gastrointestinal tract and converted to glucose in the liver. Fats and proteins, the other major nutrients, can also be converted to glucose in the liver in a process called gluconeogenesis. Thus, between meals and during times of starvation, the liver is able to maintain the blood-sugar level by conversion of protein and fat to glucose.

Within cells, tiny engines known as mitochondria produce energy for cellular activities by combining glucose with oxygen. Carbon dioxide and water are produced as by-products. Carbon dioxide is exhaled through the lungs, and water is excreted through the kidneys.

Though many organs can also produce energy by breaking down fats, the brain requires glucose. For the brain to function, the blood sugar must be maintained above a level of 50 (i.e., 50 milligrams of glucose per 100 cubic centimeters of blood plasma). Below this level, you become confused, tired, and disoriented. Very low levels can cause seizures, coma, or death.

To protect the brain, your body works to maintain a blood-sugar level over 50. In normal people in the fasting state (between meals), blood sugar is maintained between 70 and 110. Diabetes is defined as a blood-sugar level in the fasting state of more than 125.

When you eat, nutrients are absorbed from the food in your gastrointestinal tract, and glucose passes into your bloodstream. Your blood sugar rises. Between meals, your blood-sugar level is maintained by your liver, which stores excess glucose in the form of glycogen and reconverts it to glucose when needed. Glycogen stores in the liver are depleted after 24–48 hours of fasting. Then, glucose is produced by the breakdown of body proteins. The main source of energy in the fasting state, however, comes from the metabolism of stored fat, called triglycerides.

When blood sugar gets too low

When glucose levels fall, a hormone called glucagon, which, like insulin, is made in the pancreas, stimulates glucose production by the liver. The stress hormones epinephrine, norepinephrine, and cortisol also result in increased levels of blood glucose. Conditions of stress may substantially elevate the blood sugar. One other hormone, called growth hormone, has the effect of raising blood-sugar levels. Thus, there are five hormones acting at various times to keep the blood sugar from going too low, and one hormone, insulin, acting to keep it from going too high. Clearly the body recognizes the critical importance of close blood-sugar control.

During prolonged fasting, blood sugar drops significantly. Glycogen stored in the liver becomes depleted, and stores of fat in the body are used up. The liver must then use body protein to manufacture glucose, causing muscle wasting. In good health and with regular nutritious meals, the blood-sugar level stays in balance through the sensitive interaction of the regulatory hormones insulin and glucagon.

When blood sugar gets too high

The kidneys, in filtering blood to remove protein waste products, along with excess salt and water, usually absorb whatever glucose is filtered. Beyond a blood-sugar level of 150–180, however, the kidneys can no longer absorb all the filtered glucose, and it spills out and is lost in the urine.

When glucose passes into the urine, it takes other substances along with it. In this process, called osmotic diuresis, the higher the blood-sugar level, the more glucose goes into the urine—and the more other substances are lost. Many of these substances are important for proper body function, such as water, bicarbonate, calcium, magnesium, potassium, sodium, and chloride. Among the trace minerals lost are copper, zinc, manganese, molybdenum, chromium, and selenium. Though present in small amounts, these minerals are nonetheless essential for normal functioning.

Also depleted in this process are water-soluble vitamins, including vitamin C and all the B vitamins. The loss of these vitamins impairs growth, healing, immune function, cardiac and respiratory functions, thought, and memory.

Factors Contributing to High Blood Sugar (Diabetes)
• Overweight • Stress • Excessive eating of high glycemic-index foods—those that tend to rapidly raise the blood sugar (see chapter six for more information on the glycemic index) • Coexisting illness, such as infection, injury, heart attack, stroke • Steroid use • Failure to take insulin (type-1 diabetes) • Use of various medications, such as those used to control high blood pressure like diuretics and beta blockers
Factors Contributing to Low Blood Sugar
• Excessive exercise, especially if taking medication for diabetes • Failure to eat • Alcohol • Too much insulin • Too much oral blood-sugar-lowering medication • Use of beta blockers (for treating high blood pressure), which can block glucose production by the liver

These important nutrients are all lost through the kidneys as if through a sieve. They must be continually replaced. The higher the blood sugar goes and the more nutrients are lost, the harder it is to keep up.

What Insulin Does

As a hormone, insulin regulates cellular activities. Made only in the pancreas, an organ located beneath the stomach, insulin is released into the bloodstream only in very small amounts, but it is very potent. Most people produce about 40 units of insulin a day, enough to half fill a very small syringe, or about one hundredth of an ounce. The islets of Langerhans, composed of cells distributed diffusely throughout the pancreas, make insulin. These cells are called beta cells. The rest of the pancreas makes digestive enzymes that break down food in the small intestine.

When the blood sugar rises after eating, the pancreas senses this increase and releases insulin into the bloodstream. Insulin then circulates throughout the body and helps glucose move into cells, where it is broken down for energy or stored. Insulin doesn't enter into cells to do its work. Instead, it binds to an insulin receptor on the cell wall. This signals the cell to mobilize glucose transporters, which move from inside the cell to fuse with the membrane. Glucose then passes through the glucose transporter into the cell.

The mechanism for controlling blood sugar is exquisitely sensitive. If the pancreas releases too much insulin into the bloodstream, too much blood sugar will be used up, its level will drop, and the brain will suffer. This is what happens in reactive hypoglycemia, which occurs most often in young women. When their blood sugar falls too low, they feel weak, shaky, and dizzy.

If the pancreas releases too little insulin or if body cells become insensitive to normal amounts of insulin, the blood sugar goes too high, and the disease called diabetes mellitus occurs.

When factors enhance the action of insulin, you need less of the hormone to lower your blood sugar to a normal level. On the other hand, when factors block the action of insulin, you need more of it. The table on the facing page shows some insulin enhancing and blocking factors.

Juvenile Diabetes (Type 1)

Just a few years ago, doctors were able to make a clear distinction between the two different forms of diabetes—juvenile diabetes and adult-onset diabetes. In juvenile diabetes, which accounts for less than 10 percent of cases, the pancreas is damaged, losing the ability to produce the hormone insulin, which is necessary to control levels of blood sugar. As a result of the body's inability to manufacture its own insulin, those with the disease have to rely on insulin injections for the rest of their lives. There is no cure.

Although juvenile diabetes can occur in babies less than a year old, the majority of cases are found in youngsters aged 6 to 18. Fewer cases appear in adults 20 to 40, and rarely after age 40.

INSULIN ENHANCERS AND BLOCKERS

Insulin Enhancers	Insulin Blockers
Happiness	Stress
Exercise	Inactivity
Low Weight	Obesity
High-fiber diets	Low-fiber diets
Eating foods that don't raise blood sugar much (low glycemic-index foods)	Eating simple or refined carbohydrates (high glycemic-index foods)
Specific Nutrients: Magnesium B vitamins, especially biotin Chromium Vanadium Essential fatty acids Lipoic acid	Nutrient deficiencies (especially magnesium)
	Fever
	Infection
	Injury
	Hypothyroidism
	Medications: Diuretics Beta blockers

Possible Triggers of Type 1 Diabetes

Although the jury is still out regarding the cause of juvenile diabetes, the consensus of medical opinion is that its cause may be due to either a viral infection or similar stress that triggers an immune reaction. Lymphocytes, white cells forming part of the body's defense system, are misdirected. Instead of attacking a foreign invader, they turn against the body's own beta cells, islands of cells in the pancreas that make insulin. Strangely, the rest of the pancreatic cells are unaffected and continue to make digestive enzymes.

Another possibility is that antibodies against the virus may cross-react against pancreatic cells, or the virus itself may attack the pancreas. A number of other autoimmune diseases may occur simultaneously with juvenile diabetes. These include thyroiditis (inflammation of the thyroid) with hypothyroidism (loss of thyroid hormone production), adrenal insufficiency (loss of production of adrenal hormones, mainly cortisone, resulting in weakness, fatigue, and increased susceptibility to infection), pernicious anemia (a deficiency of vitamin B_{12}, causing cognitive and neurologic problems and anemia), myasthenia gravis (a muscle-wasting disease manifested by weakness and swallowing problems), and vitiligo (loss of skin pigmentation with irregular patches of whitened skin).

C-PEPTIDE AND INSULIN

In juvenile diabetes, the measurement of C-peptide (a by-product of the release of insulin) in the blood is low because there's a deficiency of insulin. In Type 2 diabetes, the C-peptide level is normal or high, since insulin is produced in excess. Because the C-peptide level reflects the production of insulin, doctors often measure it to determine the degree of insulin resistance in Type 2 diabetics. An elevated C-peptide indicates more resistance to the action of insulin. With nutritional improvements, the C-peptide level falls because less insulin is needed.

Is juvenile diabetes hereditary?

Unlike adult-onset diabetes, in which heredity plays a significant role, juvenile diabetes doesn't appear to run in families or be passed down from parent to child. Parents, siblings, and children of people with juvenile diabetics rarely get the disease. On the other hand, identical twins of juvenile diabetics do become diabetic almost half the time.

DIAGNOSING JUVENILE (TYPE-I) DIABETES

Juvenile diabetes occurs in only 10 percent of diabetics. These are some of its indicators:

- The patient is less than age 20
- The patient has no family history of diabetes
- Weight loss has been going on for several days or weeks, due to excessive loss of glucose and fluids in the urine.
- Weakness, fatigue, drowsiness, and lethargy are very common.
- Vision is often blurry

Pancreatic Damage and the Onset of Diabetes

Studies have shown that even before the outset of Type 1 diabetes, antibodies can be detected against the insulin-making cells of the pancreas. Thus, juvenile diabetics live for years with a smoldering inflammation in the pancreas, but without symptoms. Eventually, this inflammation impairs insulin production to the point that the blood sugar can no longer be controlled.

Active disease, however, does not occur until stress intervenes in the form of fever, infection, overly strenuous activity, injury, or psychological distress. At such times, stress hormones are released along with an increase in the metabolic rate, thus requiring more insulin to control the rise in the blood-sugar level. But because the pancreas is damaged, the demand for increased insulin cannot be satisfied. As the blood-sugar level progressively rises, it sets in motion the symptoms that lead to the diagnosis of Type 1 diabetes: excessive urination (with water and nutrient losses), weight loss, weakness, confusion, and altered blood chemistries.

For children already diagnosed with diabetes, stress is always a danger because of the havoc it can play with blood-sugar control. In order to prevent the serious complications that stress can trigger, it often becomes necessary to administer larger and more frequent doses of insulin.

TWO VITAMINS FOR EARLY PREVENTION

Started before the onset of illness or early in its course, nicotinamide (a form of vitamin B_3) can sometimes slow or even prevent damage to the pancreas. Nicotinamide is related to niacin but does not cause the flushing or liver inflammation that can occur with high doses of niacin. A dose of 1,500–2,000 mg a day can be given.

Also, in animal studies, vitamin D supplementation has been shown to prevent the onset of diabetes in those with a hereditary tendency to develop it (*Prevention*, December 1999).

Insulin Administration

Insulin is always required in the treatment of Type 1 diabetes. It is ineffective when given orally and must always be given in an injection. Insulin was once obtained from beef and pork pancreatic tissue. Since this kind of insulin is different from human insulin, allergic reactions sometimes occurred and antibodies formed that reduced the insulin's effectiveness. Now, through the marvel of genetic technology, insulin is produced by bacteria with a structure identical to that of human insulin.

Insulin is available in short- and long-acting formulations. A new insulin called lispro begins to work within minutes after injection. Short- and long-acting insulins are often injected together before a meal to control the blood-sugar elevation that occurs after eating and to provide blood-sugar regulation throughout the day. The most effective blood-sugar control occurs when insulin is given before each meal. Some patients, especially those on optimal dietary programs, can take insulin less often with good blood-sugar control.

Insulin is sometimes prescribed for Type 2 diabetes, when oral medications fail to work. The use of insulin can often be prevented in those people with proper dietary management, exercise, weight loss, and nutritional supplements.

The honeymoon period

After diabetes has been diagnosed by the measurement of an abnormally elevated blood-sugar level, a "honeymoon" phase often occurs. During this period, the blood sugar returns to normal or near normal while using little or no insulin. It is thought that this honeymoon phase represents a partial recovery of pancreatic insulin production. I believe it is also due to the relief of a stressful situation and the institution of improved dietary practices. For instance, eliminating refined sugar from the diet would certainly lead to the need for less insulin.

The honeymoon period can last anywhere from a month to a year, during which time one's insulin requirements are minimal. This is only true for juvenile diabetes. There is no honeymoon period in adult-onset diabetes.

After beginning rigorous diets with high doses of supplements, I have frequently seen young patients not require insulin for extended periods. Subsequently, insulin will become necessary, but the dosage is minimized with exercise, weight control, good food choices, and the addition of vitamins and minerals.

Insulin alone is not enough

If you get nothing else from this book, let it be the understanding that depending on insulin alone to manage juvenile diabetes is an inadequate approach. Unless a lifestyle program is adopted, insulin alone will not provide satisfactory blood-sugar control. Blood-sugar levels can go too high or too low; energy can all but disappear. Vision can get cloudy, and mood can fluctuate. The dose of insulin that handles the blood sugar after a high-protein meal will not be adequate for a meal of concentrated carbohydrates. The lower the dose of insulin that is needed, the less chance there is of a low blood-sugar reaction.

Superimposed illness and infection also require higher doses of insulin because during these episodes, the blood sugar will rise. A day without exercise raises the blood sugar and requires more insulin, even if the diet is unchanged. Parents with children who do not understand the need for consistency in dietary choices will see blood-sugar levels going up and down like a yo-yo, even though the insulin is given consistently. Keep in mind that treatment succeeds best with the lifestyle modifications of diet, exercise, weight control, and nutritional supplementation that are discussed in this book. Make the commitment to following a complete program every day. The closer it is followed, the fewer the daily problems and the better the long-term prognosis.

Outlook for Juvenile Diabetes

Diabetic complications are not inevitable. Many people with juvenile diabetes do not develop kidney, eye, nerve, or cardiovascular diseases, even after decades of managing diabetes.

- Visual deficits can improve.
- Neuropathy (nerve damage) is reversible. It can improve.
- Cardiovascular disease is reversible. It can improve.
- Kidney disease is not reversible, but it can be stabilized or slowed down if addressed early enough.
- In all cases it is easier and more desirable to prevent complications than to handle them once they have started.

To prevent and treat diabetic complications, you must:

1. Control blood sugar.
2. Supplement with specific vitamins, minerals, and antioxidants (see chapter 7).
3. Maintain ideal weight.
4. Exercise.
5. Reduce stress.
6. Avoid toxins, including trans-fatty acids, pesticides, herbicides, food additives and preservatives, and heavy metals.
7. Correct other disease-intensifying factors, especially high blood pressure, high cholesterol, high triglycerides, and high homocysteine—a cardiovascular risk factor detected in the blood (see below).

Preventing cardiovascular disease

Eighty percent of deaths in diabetics are due to cardiovascular disease. This is caused by atherosclerosis, the depositing of cholesterol and other fats in and along the walls of arteries throughout the body. These deposits cause an inflammatory reaction, with white blood cells releasing chemicals that damage the arteries. Calcium is also deposited. Eventually, these blood vessels close off, or a deposit ruptures into the blood vessel and initiates the formation of a blood clot. If this occurs in the heart, the blockage of an artery causes the death of cardiac tissue—otherwise known as a heart attack. If this occurs in the brain, nerve tissue is damaged and a stroke occurs, often with paralysis of an arm or leg.

The elevated blood sugar in diabetics causes direct damage to artery walls, making them more susceptible to further damage caused by high blood pressure, high cholesterol, high triglycerides, and high homocysteine. The most effective way to prevent cardiovascular disease is to control all of these factors. Fortunately, the same lifestyle changes that control diabetes are effective in lowering blood pressure, cholesterol and triglycerides:

- High blood pressure improves with weight loss, exercise, reduced stress, reduction of salt intake, and increased intake of magnesium and potassium. The sodium (salt) content of fast foods and packaged foods is much higher than that of whole foods such as vegetables and fruits. Vegetables and fruits are also very high in magnesium and potassium.
- High cholesterol and triglycerides decline with blood-sugar control, exercise, weight loss, and restricting high glycemic-index (high sugar) and high-fat foods.
- Homocysteine levels can be lowered by taking vitamin B supplements. Homocysteine is a protein measured in the blood that contributes to atherosclerosis. Its origin is dietary protein. It can also become elevated due to genetic factors or kidney disease. To lower homocysteine levels, take the following: vitamin B_6, up to 500 mg a day (discuss this with your physician as too high a dose can cause toxicity); folic acid, 1–5 mg per day; and vitamin B_{12}, 1,000–2,500 mg per day.

All of these factors are modifiable. Although diabetics are subject to cardiovascular events, my program offers a substantial reduction of risk. Insulin alone is not the answer. Dietary changes, weight control, exercise, and targeted nutritional supplements provided under the guidance of a knowledgeable medical professional can be extremely effective in avoiding unwanted complications.

Adult-Onset (Type 2) Diabetes

Adult-onset or Type 2 diabetes occurs primarily in overweight adults over age 40 who often have a family history of the disease. It has nothing to do with the pancreatic damage or insulin deficiency that is found in Type 1 diabetes. Instead, it arises from insulin resistance, which is a consequence of the following lifestyle factors:

- Obesity
- Lack of exercise
- Eating high glycemic-index foods (foods high in sugar or refined carbohydrates that elevate blood sugar and require increasing amounts of insulin to lower it)
- Lack of necessary nutrients, particularly magnesium, chromium, essential fatty acids, lipoic acid, and vanadium

Other factors that interfere with the action of insulin include stress, infection, trauma, and the use of certain drugs, especially steroids.

Because the pancreas is functioning properly and producing insulin, adult-onset diabetes is also referred to as non-insulin-dependent diabetes mellitus (NIDDM). Despite the production of insulin, problems occur because the body has lost its ability to respond to insulin. It is a state of insulin resistance, where the above factors prevent insulin from exerting its blood-sugar-lowering effect.

Unlike in Type 1 diabetes, where there is a reduced production of insulin (not insulin resistance), in Type 2 diabetes, insulin levels are normal or high. Like juvenile (insulin-dependent) diabetes, this form of the disease can also be controlled through diet, exercise, attainment of ideal weight, and the use of nutritional supplements. Unlike insulin-dependent diabetes, this form of the disease is reversible. It often can be cured.

The Type 2 diabetes paradox

In adult-onset diabetes, natural insulin levels are high, so that administering insulin only *worsens* the situation by increasing fat deposits and aggravating obesity. The reason insulin increases fat deposits is because its metabolic action involves the transformation of sugar into fat within the cells. Insulin is a fat-producing and fat-storing hormone. It allows the body to store energy as fat, to be used during times when food is not available. Insulin works against us, however, when it is produced in excess. Then it causes more fat to be deposited in the body and makes us obese. This creates even more insulin resistance and reinforces a vicious cycle: insulin causes obesity, which creates more insulin resistance, so we give more insulin and cause more obesity.

Adult-Onset Diabetes Affects Children Too

Thanks to the fattening of Americans of all ages, it is no longer possible to make clear-cut distinctions based on age with regard to diabetes. Adult-onset diabetes now affects an increasing percentage of young people still in their teens and twenties. Therefore, adult-onset diabetes is now more correctly referred to as Type 2, non-insulin-dependent diabetes, and juvenile diabetes as Type 1, insulin-dependent diabetes.

People who are overweight, don't exercise or perform physical work, eat large amounts of sugars and simple carbohydrates, and have diets deficient in certain vitamins, minerals, and essential fatty acids are at risk to develop insulin resistance, which leads to Type 2 diabetes. When a factor such as weight gain causes insulin resistance, the pancreas has to release larger amounts of insulin to return the blood sugar to a normal level. As the weight goes up, insulin resistance increases and more insulin must be released.

As the weight gain continues, however, insulin resistance increases to the point that the pancreas cannot produce enough insulin to maintain the blood sugar at normal levels. Thus, even though the insulin level is elevated, the blood sugar still goes up. The pancreas has used up its reserves and cannot produce insulin at a higher rate. After years of worsening insulin resistance, diabetes finally occurs. The pancreas of some Type 2 diabetics eventually seems to give out, and insulin is required. Such people may actually have a late-occurring form of Type 1 diabetes. But for practical purposes, it can be assumed that Type 2 diabetes is reversible at all ages, even in people in their 70s and 80s. With help, the disease can be eliminated in young people, since they can more easily adapt to the lifestyle changes necessary for a cure.

Type 2 Diabetes in Children: An Emerging Epidemic

Physicians like Dr. Robin S. Goland, co-director of the Naomi Barrie Diabetes Center at Columbia University's College of Physicians and Surgeons, are reporting that 10 to 20 percent of new pediatric patients have Type 2 diabetes, compared to less than 4 percent just five years ago.

"Ten years ago we were teaching medical students that you didn't see this disease in people under 40," she says. "Now we're seeing it in people under 10. With the numbers we are starting to see, this could be the beginning of an epidemic."

Goland's observations are born out by research at the University of Cincinnati College of Medicine Diabetes Center, where a recent study found that from 1984 to 1992, the percentage of children with Type 2 diabetes increased from 2 to 4 percent. By 1994, that number increased to 16 percent—a remarkable four-fold increase.

Clinical observations from pediatricians and others who treat many young people support these studies. In 1998, Dr. Kenneth L. Jones of the University of California at San Diego said that during the previous five years, local area clinics reported a tenfold increase in the number of childhood Type 2 diabetes.

At present, there's no routine screening of children for subclinical (without symptoms) diabetes. Such screening needs to be done, especially for children who are overweight or have a family history of diabetes.

Diagnosing Type 2 Diabetes

Nine out of ten diabetics have Type 2, a condition of insulin resistance, not a deficiency of production. Type 2 diabetes is usually diagnosed by the following factors:

- Patient is generally age 40 or older (though this is changing, as you can see from the statistics above).
- Patient is overweight or has a good-sized paunch (i.e., a large band of abdominal fat).
- Young patients are generally obese and inactive.
- A strong family history of diabetes is present.
- The C-peptide blood level is high, indicating greater than normal insulin production and the presence of an insulin-resistant state.
- Diabetes often reveals itself during infection or stress (see box below).
- Diabetes may occur during use of steroids.
- Ketoacidosis, a condition that impairs the regulation of many body functions, rarely occurs. Ketoacidosis is much more prevalent in Type 1 diabetes.

The First Symptoms of Type 2 Diabetes

Because its symptoms often take years to become health-threatening, people tend to feel that Type 2 diabetes is less severe than Type 1. But if Type 2 diabetes goes undiagnosed or is left untreated, damage to blood vessels can result in life-threatening complications in 10 to 20 years. Unlike Type 1 diabetes, which rapidly produces serious symptoms leading to early diagnosis, Type 2 diabetes can smolder undetected for years, silently causing progressive vascular damage. The first clue to the presence of Type 2 diabetes may be the occurrence of neuropathy (pain or numbness in the extremities, usually in the feet or legs) or visual loss, which on further evaluation leads to the detection of an elevated blood-sugar level. By that time, damage may already have occurred that cannot be repaired.

The Role of Genetics

Genetics plays a larger role in Type 2 than in Type 1 diabetes. About 40 percent of siblings and 30 percent of children of Type 2 diabetics develop insulin resistance leading to diabetes. In identical twins, if one has Type 2 diabetes, the other will almost certainly be affected.

In the September 1999 issue of *Diabetes*, researchers reported discovering the first gene associated with the kind of insulin resistance that occurs in Type 2 diabetes. This gene is responsible for the production of a protein that blocks insulin from enabling glucose to enter cells. Researchers hope this discovery will help them prevent production of this protein. Even so, this would only help some of the people with insulin resistance. Others, who don't have the gene, may also be insulin resistant, raising the possibility that other genes may also be involved.

ARE YOU AT RISK?

Certain people are at higher risk of developing Type 2 diabetes. These include:

- African-Americans, Latinos, and Native Americans (who are up to 10 times higher at risk)
- Infants with either very low or very high birth weights
- Children whose mothers were malnourished during pregnancy
- Those with high blood pressure, heart disease, and certain cancers
- Children whose parents have Type 2 diabetes

Preventing Long-Term Complications

Why is it important to learn and follow this program? There are scary statistics related to the long-term complications of diabetes, the same statistics that physicians recite to their patients in order to compel urgency and compliance. Up to one third of all diabetics ultimately develop kidney failure. The incidence of blindness in diabetics is 20 times higher than in the general population. Neurologic impairment is common. There is a significant risk of premature death due to cardiovascular events. Amputation may occur due to diminished peripheral circulation.

The good news is that because such complications require years to develop, they can be prevented by managing the disease correctly. Study after study in the last few years validates the fact that these complications are preventable. They are preventable by following the right diet, taking the right supplements, exercising, and maintaining the proper weight. They are preventable by avoiding toxins, cigarettes, alcohol, and artificial foods. Most important of all is maintaining an unyielding optimism and learning to handle setbacks and make necessary changes.

Hypoglycemia

Hypoglycemia means low blood sugar. Because the brain's major source of energy is glucose, low blood sugar deprives the brain of fuel, causing fatigue, jitteriness, loss of concentration, confusion, tremor, or agitation. Very low levels can cause seizures, coma, or permanent brain damage.

In diabetics, hypoglycemia is due to excessive doses of insulin or oral diabetic medications. It may also occur when insulin or medication is taken without eating, or with too small a meal. Exercise may also cause hypoglycemia by increasing the effect of diabetic medication. This is because exercise promotes the entry of glucose into the cells, independent of the action of insulin, thus lowering the blood sugar.

In non-diabetics, hypoglycemia occurs with fasting, usually for more than 12 hours. Another condition, called reactive hypoglycemia, occurs one or two hours after eating foods with a high glycemic index, such as candy bars or soft drinks. These foods rapidly elevate the blood sugar. Insulin is then released in excess, causing blood-sugar depression.

Alcohol, when taken without food, prevents the liver from producing glucose and can cause severe and life-threatening hypoglycemia in both diabetics and non-diabetics. When a diabetic has a change in mental status, it may be due to either low or very high blood sugar. A simple test of blood sugar gives the answer.

Diabetic ketoacidosis

Ketoacidosis occurs only when insulin is deficient, and is therefore not seen in Type 1 diabetes. High blood sugar results in increased urine volume with loss of water and salt. Dehydration occurs. Low insulin, along with high levels of another pancreatic hormone called glucagon, causes the release of fatty acids from body tissues. In the liver the fatty acids convert to ketones, creating an acid state in the body called acidosis. Acidosis impairs the regulation of many body functions, including the balance of potassium and magnesium.

The combination of high blood sugar, dehydration, and acidosis causes rapidly progressive weakness, confusion, and loss of consciousness. It can be fatal. Intensive therapy with intravenous insulin and balanced fluids usually resolves this condition without residual effects. Regular monitoring of blood sugar in insulin-dependent diabetics should prevent ketoacidosis from occurring.

Other complications

Diabetic complications occur when blood sugar is poorly controlled. The more closely the blood sugar is controlled, the less likely is the occurrence of the following complications of the kidneys, eye, nerves, and cardiovascular system:

Retinopathy: Damage to the part of the eye called the retina, which receives visual information and transmits it to the brain. It includes damage caused by bleeding, leakage of fluid, and proliferation of excessive numbers of new blood vessels. There is scarring and progressive loss of vision. It is often treated by laser photocoagulation, cauterizing the leaky blood vessels.

Organ damage: In diabetes, changes in protein function caused by high blood glucose may damage organs. Glucose combines with various proteins to form AGES—advanced glycosylation end products. These end products alter the normal protein structure and impair function in many different organs (the most vulnerable are the cardiovascular system, kidneys, eyes and nerves). The higher the blood sugar, the more AGES are formed. Normalizing a high blood sugar will reduce the level of AGES by 40 percent in one week.

High blood pressure: Many diabetics develop high blood pressure. It is often the result of overweight, high salt intake, and a lack of exercise. High blood pressure greatly increases the risk of heart attack and stroke, and causes rapid progression of diabetic kidney disease. When kidney disease occurs, it is responsible for further blood-pressure elevation. Thus, kidney disease causes high blood pressure, which causes more kidney disease—a vicious cycle leading to kidney failure. High blood pressure can be controlled with medication, but it can also be controlled with weight loss, reduced salt intake, and exercise.

Low blood pressure: This occurs in diabetics as a consequence of damage to the nerves that regulate blood-vessel tone. When you stand up, blood settles into your legs. The blood pressure is maintained, however, by increased contraction within blood vessel walls.

When these nerves are damaged, blood pressure falls when you stand. There is not enough pressure to provide blood to the brain. Weakness, dizziness, or falls can occur. Low blood pressure also commonly occurs when high blood pressure is overtreated with medication. In diabetics who have nerve damage, it is important to measure the standing blood pressure and to reduce blood pressure medication if the standing pressure is low.

Peripheral vascular disease: In diabetics, blood vessels to the arms and especially the legs may become narrowed by cholesterol and calcium deposits, as well as by thickening and tightening of smooth muscle within the blood vessel. Because the blood supply is reduced, hands and feet become cool and discolored, and may develop ulcers that cannot heal. There is pain and weakness in the legs (claudication) with walking, which is alleviated with rest. However, this is a difficult condition to treat because medication is often ineffective. Surgical therapy, including vascular balloon dilatation and surgical bypass, is dangerous and often ineffective. Alternative therapies including chelation (a nonsurgical treatment that improves circulation by ridding the body of excess toxins, especially metals), hyperbaric oxygen (oxygen delivered under high pressure in enclosed metal chambers), or special leg-pressure devices are often helpful.

Peripheral vascular disease is a late occurrence in diabetes that often indicates severe and generalized hardening of the arteries throughout the body. It occurs as well in non-diabetics, especially those who smoke. Smoking invariably worsens peripheral vascular disease in diabetics, and must be stopped to prevent eventual amputation.

Cardiac and cerebrovascular disease: Eighty percent of deaths in diabetics are due to heart disease and stroke. Atherosclerlosis occurs at an accelerated rate in diabetics due to the damage caused to arteries by elevated blood sugar as well as the greater frequency in diabetics of other risk factors, including high cholesterol and triglycerides, high blood pressure, and increased blood coagulation. Atherosclerosis affects all the blood vessels in the body, but its effects occur predominantly in the heart and brain. Heart attacks can cause sudden death. Recurrent heart attacks, or progressive damage to the small blood vessels (microvasculature) of the heart, can result in weakening of the heart muscle, called cardiomyopathy. This can lead to congestive heart failure, when the heart is too weak to pump blood effectively to the rest of the body. Congestive heart failure is the major cause of hospitalization for people over 65 in this country. Over time, this condition may fail to respond to medication, and death follows.

A new therapy called enhanced external counterpulsation (EECP)™ holds promise for cardiac patients. Inflatable cuffs are wrapped around the legs and pelvis. When inflated with air during the relaxation phase of the cardiac cycle (diastole), the cuffs force blood up the aorta back into the heart. This pulsatile flow of blood dilates the coronary arteries and causes new blood vessels to be formed. It is a non-surgical way of treating coronary artery disease and possibly improving congestive heart failure.

A stroke is a form of brain damage that is caused by the occlusion (obstruction or closure) of a blood vessel in the brain and less often by hemorrhage. Heart attacks and strokes often occur in the same individuals, because both are caused by the same process—atherosclerosis. Strokes may cause paralysis of an arm, leg, or one side of the face, or an impairment of speech or cognition.

Atherosclerosis is a progressive disorder. It often begins early in life, even during the teenage years, but usually does not cause perceptible injury until after age 50. It is important to remember that atherosclerosis is reversible, that the damage to blood vessels can be halted and repaired, using the same lifestyle changes described in this book for treating diabetes.

COMPLICATIONS FROM BOTH TYPE 1 AND TYPE 2 DIABETES

Most of these diabetic complications are directly related to the degree of blood-sugar elevation and develop over many years:

Eyes
Retinopathy (damage to the part of the eye called the retina)
Cataracts
Blindness
Kidneys
Protein loss
Renal failure
Nerves
Numbness, tingling, burning, pains in hands and feet
Nerve damage (neuropathy)
Muscle wasting
Paralysis of arms and legs
Gastrointestinal nerve damage with bloating, vomiting, diarrhea, and constipation
Bladder paralysis
Cardiovascular
Low blood pressure
High blood pressure, high cholesterol
Atherosclerosis
Heart attack
Heart failure
Stroke (damage to brain tissue due to lack of blood supply)
Peripheral vascular disease (insufficient blood supply to hands and feet due to arteriosclerosis), gangrene, amputation
Skin
Hard-to-heal infections and ulcers

The Outlook for Type 2 Diabetes

A Type 1 diabetic will always be a diabetic, although the situation can be greatly eased. A Type 2 diabetic, however, can be cured, and medication can be eliminated. Blood-sugar levels can become normalized if:

- Exercise becomes a consistent part of daily life. Exercise enables glucose to enter cells independent of insulin action. In effect, this means that exercise itself lowers the blood sugar, without the need for insulin.
- The diabetic loses weight, thus enhancing insulin activity. Obesity, on the other hand, impedes the action of insulin, creating insulin resistance.
- Foods high in protein, fiber, and whole grains become the mainstay of the diet. They do not cause the blood sugar to rise after eating as much as simple sugars and refined carbohydrates.
- Nutritional supplements are taken to enhance the action of insulin.

The Drug Approach: Type 1

Traditional diabetic care focuses on the choice and proper use of either insulin or oral agents, or both. For the insulin-dependent (Type 1) diabetic, the emphasis is on:

- Type of insulin—whether long-, short-, or ultra-short acting
- Schedule of insulin administration
- Coordination of meals
- Blood-sugar testing with drug dosing

Even when the patient is on insulin, oral drugs are frequently added to "smooth out" blood-sugar control.

I have personally seen doctors start diabetic patients on one drug, switch to a second because their blood-sugar levels remained elevated, and move on to a third drug when they still showed no improvement. This single-minded focus on drugs is a shortsighted and regrettable approach that reflects the restricted training offered to physicians. It also reflects the excessive influence of the pharmaceutical industry on medical decision making.

Emphasizing drug treatment for Type 1 diabetes can actually retard progress. By adding proper nutrition and exercise to the therapy, blood sugar can be stabilized and insulin reduced. Yet diabetic children and their parents are often denied this information because the physician doesn't consider it important enough, or doesn't have time to explain it, or doesn't understand it himself. Even the dietician who instructs the family may offer the wrong recommendations.

Type 1 diabetes is not just an insulin-deficient state that is treatable simply by providing insulin. It requires attention to a number of factors, including nutrition, supplements, exercise, stressors, and the family support system. The physician who does not offer comprehensive support is shortchanging his patient and offering inferior care.

The Drug Approach: Type 2

In order to regulate blood sugar in Type 2 diebetes, physicians individualize treatment with one or a combination of drugs from the following classes of medications:

1. Sulfonylureas—these stimulate the pancreas to produce more insulin. This is the oldest class of oral agents. It fails to work in 20% of patients (primary failure) and loses effectiveness in patients who initially respond, at the rate of 5% to 10% per year. Hypoglycemia is a common side effect. Type 2 diabetics typically manifest excess insulin production, since the pancreas is working overtime to overcome insulin resistance. Sulfonylureas (SUs) further increase insulin levels. Since insulin production is an independent risk factor for cardiovascular disease, these drugs may increase the risk of heart disease and stroke.
2. Biguanides—these reduce glucose production by the liver. Only metformin is now available. It does not cause hypoglycemia, but can cause nausea and loss of appetite. It may rarely cause lactic acidosis, a very serious metabolic

disorder. It should not be employed in those with liver or kidney disease, heart failure, or alcohol abuse.

3. Alpha-glucosidase inhibitors—these block the enzymes that digest complex carbohydrates in the gastrointestinal tract. The glucose-lowering effect is mild. Side effects are gas, bloating, and diarrhea.

4. Thiazolidinediones—these enhance the activity of insulin. Rezulin, the drug recently banned for causing fatal liver damage, was the first drug introduced in this class. There are two remaining drugs in this group considered safer for the liver. These drugs, however, cause weight gain, already a major problem for Type 2 diabetics.

5. Benzoic acid derivatives—these stimulate insulin secretion in a manner similar to the sulfonylureas and are less likely to cause hypoglycemia.

6. Insulin—this is mainly used by Type 2 diabetics who are non-obese, younger, severely hyperglycemic, or pregnant. It is also often used at times of stress, such as surgery, infections, or accidents.

Drug Dangers

Drugs are taken more often to relieve symptoms than to save lives. Ironically, the symptoms they relieve are often replaced by new symptoms they create. *The Physicians' Desk Reference* lists paragraphs and sometimes pages of drug complications. Antibiotics cause diarrhea; anti-inflammatories cause gastrointestinal bleeding; antidepressants cause constipation, urinary retention, and dry mouth. Sleeping pills cause confusion, memory loss, lack of coordination, and falls. Combinations of drugs for multiple problems cause multiple complications.

SIDE EFFECTS FROM DIABETES DRUGS

Did you know that the side effects of commonly prescribed diabetes medications can cause dizziness, hunger, fatigue, and other symptoms of hypoglycemia?

In a survey of 500 patients with Type 2 diabetes, only

16% realized that their oral anti-diabetic drug had side effects, although 72% of these respondents were taking sulfonylurea (SU), a class of conventional drugs that may induce hypoglycemia. Common symptoms reported by these patients included weakness, fatigue, anxiety, nervousness, sweating, and impaired vision. Uncontrollable hunger, another common side effect, was reported by 18% of SU patients, while 26% felt they had gained weight within the first few months after starting their diabetes medication. One out of five surveyed felt that their quality of life had suffered since beginning their SU therapies. They reported such emotional factors as a decreased sense of well-being, feelings of hopelessness in managing their diabetes, and an impaired social life.

Are these drugs really effective or do you need another drug for the drugs' side effects? Clearly, drugs alone are not the answer. Modifications in diet and exercise can give you the power to manage your diabetes without sacrificing well-being and without dependence on drugs.

(Source: The Diabetes Control and Complications Trial Research Group. "The Effect of Intensive Treatment of Diabetes on the Development and Progression of Long-Term Complications in Insulin-Dependent Diabetes Mellitus." *New England Journal of Medicine* 1993. 329:977–986.)

In recent years, we have been hearing more and more about drugs with life-shortening effects that counteract their benefits. About 108,000 people die yearly in hospitals as a consequence of adverse drug effects, making this the fifth greatest cause of death in the United States. Another 90,000 deaths a year occur as a result of therapeutic errors, such as misdiagnosis, improper prescribing, or poor advice. Thus, we have 200,000 deaths a year occurring not as a result of illness, but because of the medical treatment that is provided.

The sad irony is that drugs intended to save lives frequently take lives. For example, the FDA bans several drugs every year because of "excessive deaths." Some drugs used in cancer therapy can suppress the immune system and permit a lethal infection to develop. Other drugs used to treat irregular heart rhythms seem as likely to make people ill as to save them. According to some recent studies, calcium channel blockers have increased cardiac death rates despite having lowered blood pressure. One of the worst examples of this problem occurred recently with the diabetic drug, Rezulin.

Rezulin: A Cautionary Tale

Rezulin is a drug that can have a potent effect on blood sugar. It increases both insulin production and utilization, and has been employed in treating people with either Type 1 or Type 2 diabetes. But after the deaths of more than 60 people who suffered liver failure from this drug, Rezulin has been withdrawn from the market.

The FDA approved Rezulin for use in the United States, even though Great Britain banned this drug because of proven liver toxicity. Parke-Davis, the manufacturer, earned almost $2 billion in sales. At one point, the National Institutes of Health allocated millions of dollars toward the study of Rezulin's effectiveness in preventing Type 2 diabetes. The rationale seemed to be that it was preferable to use a drug to prevent disease than to wait to treat the disease after it developed. This was dangerous thinking, not only because it promoted a drug with dangerous complications, but also because it ignored what we know about the causes of Type 2 diabetes: obesity, inactivity, and unwise dietary choices. In fact, the only successful way to prevent this disease is by addressing these causes with lifestyle changes.

As the Rezulin body count rose, physicians were cautioned to perform frequent blood tests to detect early liver toxicity. Unfortunately, these precautions were ineffective because liver damage was rapidly progressive and fatal. Finally, Dr. Robert Misbin, the FDA physician involved in the initial approval of Rezulin, proclaimed it unsafe and requested that it be taken off the market. But not to worry. Two other drugs with similar modes of action—Actos and Avandia—stand ready to replace Rezulin. Time will tell if they are safer.

In the last three years, seven drugs have been removed from circulation because of lethal side effects. It is obvious that initial testing does not guarantee the long-term safety of a drug. Yet physicians are quick to prescribe new agents, seemingly unaware that the primary responsibility to their patient is to "Do No Harm."

I remember another diabetic drug that was banned about 30 years ago. It was called phenformin, and it caused numerous deaths from lactic acidosis, a severe acid-base disturbance. Ten years ago, phenformin returned in a different formulation, called Glucophage. Glucophage is safer and it is popular, but it can still cause fatal acidosis in patients with pre-existing kidney disease. It should only be taken by those with normal kidney function. Still, I have seen several patients with kidney problems taking this drug because their physicians were ignorant of the risk.

There are no risks involved in eliminating sugars and refined carbohydrates from the diet. There are no risks in avoiding bread, pasta, potatoes, ice cream, soft drinks, and cold cereals. No risks are incurred by never smoking cigarettes, drinking alcohol, or taking recreational drugs. There are no risks involved in the judicious use of targeted nutritional supplements.

Our treatment programs must be aligned with our intentions. We should endeavor to offer programs that are at once the safest and the most effective. Such programs already exist. They are called dietary counseling, vitamin and mineral supplementation, regular exercise, maintenance of ideal weight, and control of stress. Our health professionals should be as adept in offering these treatments as they are in prescribing drugs.

The shortsighted reliance on drugs is a learned response, one that we and our children will pay dearly for in the future. The idea that the answer to a problem lies in a bottle of pills only promotes the acquisition of more and more bottles of pills. I prefer a different answer: We must develop the determination to create a strong spirit and a resilient body that will stand up against the pharmaceutical Trojan horse. If you support your mind and body, you will need fewer drugs.

Drugs are like the gift of fire. Used with discrimination, they can be beneficial. Used carelessly, they can burn down your house and the fields around it.

Start Low, Go Slow:
The Right Approach to Drugs

When doctors need to know what dosage of a drug to prescribe, they usually look it up in the *Physicians' Desk Reference* (PDR). The PDR gets this information from the drug manufacturers. An associate professor of psychiatry at the University of California at San Diego claims that the recommended dosages for many drugs are too high, causing an array of side effects and even untimely deaths. Dr. Jay S. Cohen published his report in the Fall 1999 issue of *Postgraduate Medicine:* "Weight, age, and sex are determinants of dosage. What is not taken into account is how two people of the same weight, age, and sex can react differently to the same dose of the same drug."

According to Dr. David Bates, an associate professor of medicine at the Harvard Medical School, "In the elderly . . . it's quite clear that you get in trouble if you use a 'one size fits all' dosing, which doctors have tended to do. It may well be for younger people, too, that there's considerable variability in the way drugs are broken down."

According to Dr. Bates, physicians are taught to "start low, go slow," when prescribing drugs for older patients. He thinks that advice should apply to younger patients also.

The Challenge of Diabetes

It is a shock to learn that one's child has diabetes. Without prior knowledge of this disease and how to manage it, parents may be concerned about their ability to care for their youngster as well as the youngster's ability to care for him- or herself. Parents will need to learn how to perform needle pricks, read blood-sugar tests, administer insulin injections, watch for signs of reactions like hypogylcemia, and make sure their child eats at the right time. They will need to teach these things to their child as well. Add to that the challenge of modifying diet, adding supplements (believe it or not, most physicians still do not prescribe supplements to their diabetic patients), and upping the amount of daily exercise, all of which are critical to the management of both Type 1 and Type 2 diabetes, and families have a lot of work on their hands. But with patience and careful attention to the program, the majority of families and diabetics master the regimen so that the child is able to lead a healthy, happy, productive life.

CHAPTER 2

Diabetes Is a Family Affair

Having a child with diabetes is scary. Many children are quite ill when their diabetes is first diagnosed, and physicians are likely to emphasize how serious the situation is in order to achieve patient compliance. Families must make immediate changes in eating and exercise patterns. Repeated needle sticks, worries about high and low blood-sugar levels, and anticipation of problems contribute to the tension. Parents now fear for their children's future. "What if my child goes blind?" a parent asks. Another wonders, "Will my daughter experience kidney failure? The doctor says if she doesn't follow the program, she could get sick and die."

Q. How did my child get diabetes?
A. The cause of Type 1, or juvenile, diabetes is unclear. It may result from a viral infection triggering an autoimmune reaction against the insulin-producing cells of the pancreas.

In the case of Type 2 diabetes, the body's insulin resistance is triggered by a combination of genetic and lifestyle factors such as obesity, lack of exercise, improper food choices, and nutritional deficiencies.

Q. Will my other children get diabetes?
A. That is very unlikely. Type 1, or juvenile, diabetes rarely runs in families.

Q. Will my child die from this?
A. No. Serious complications of diabetes occur after many years and are related to insufficient blood-sugar control.

Q. Can it go away?
A. No. Juvenile diabetes is a permanent condition. Adult-onset diabetes (Type 2), however, is reversible. Type 2 diabetes in children is also reversible. These children are always overweight and underactive, and lifestyle changes can eliminate the factors causing the disease.

Q. Must my child take insulin?
A. Yes. Juvenile diabetes (Type 1) is an insulin-deficient condition. Altering the diet, exercising, maintaining ideal weight, and taking specific supplements can lower the necessary dose of insulin, but some dose of insulin is necessary.

In the case of Type 2 diabetes, making such changes can reduce the amount of insulin one needs or eliminate it entirely.

Q. What about all these finger sticks?
A. Finger-stick sugar determinations are important in determining the required dose of insulin and preventing unexpected fluctuations. If a pattern of good blood-sugar control can be established, fewer finger-stick determinations may be necessary. A machine will be available soon that can measure the blood sugar through the skin, without performing a needle stick.

Q. What if my child won't accept this?
A. Your child needs to understand what is happening. His understanding will lead to acceptance and cooperation. He also needs your unlimited support and love. He should never be blamed for his illness.

Q. Will my child be accepted by other children?
A. Children can be understanding or they can be cruel, just like adults. If your child offers the attitude that managing diabetes is just a condition of his life and explains what his situation is about, he is unlikely to be an object of derision.

Gaining Control

If your child is diagnosed with diabetes, try to learn all you can about this disease and how it relates to your child. Talk to your doctor. Read books that have a level of medical terminology you can easily follow (for some suggestions, see the Recommended Reading section at the end of this book). Don't be disturbed by conflicting information from different sources. You will gradually learn what is true in your child's situation and what works for him or her. To accomplish this, the entire family needs to become involved so that everyone is informed. Knowledge and shared responsibilities prevent misunderstandings and resentment.

Diabetic children should never be made to feel guilty for a situation they did not cause. Their problem should never be translated to an inconvenience for the family.

How Fear Paralyzes Learning

Sometimes the gut-wrenching fear that their child has a serious chronic illness they don't understand but must somehow learn to control can disturb parents so much that the learning process is paralyzed. These fears can prevent parents from acting in the best interests of their child because doing so means taking risks. That's what happened to Larry's parents when they came to our clinic and heard about a dramatically different approach to treating his diabetes.

Larry's parents loved their son and wanted him to thrive. But they were also terribly alarmed at what they perceived as upsetting the applecart, wobbly as it was, by trying a radically different approach to the management of diabetes. They had experienced enormous anxiety at the onset of their son's illness. It had taken great dedication to establish a workable program and to guide Larry in adjusting to his situation. There had been a constant fear of severe reactions and hospitalization. Having to wake up in the middle of the night to test Larry's blood sugar kept his mother perpetually tired. Yet there was some comfort in this program. Because the parents knew what to expect, the problems had become predictable.

When I suggested making changes in Larry's diet and life-style, his parents initially felt frightened and agitated. I explained that replacing the sugar and other simple carbohydrates he was eating with complex carbohydrates and more fiber would allow for improved blood-sugar control. Eating whole grains like buckwheat and oatmeal wouldn't raise Larry's blood sugar as much as simple carbohydrates like processed breakfast cereals. As a result, less insulin would be needed to prevent excessive blood-sugar elevations after eating. This in turn would eliminate the blood-sugar roller coaster that Larry was experiencing.

I explained that diabetics are more susceptible to diseases than other people because diabetes increases the rate of tissue deterioration. Diabetics are at greater risk of having heart attacks, strokes, and cataracts at earlier ages than non-diabetics. That's why it is particularly important for diabetics to eliminate unhealthy foods and food additives (such as preservatives, colorings, trans-fatty acids, and excessive salt) that have been linked to disease. Other factors that lead to illness are also especially dangerous to diabetics. For instance, cigarettes greatly increase vascular damage in diabetics, leading to heart attacks and heart failure, strokes, and leg amputations. Habits that reduce the quality of life for many people may produce catastrophic illness in diabetics. That is the reason I urge diabetics to avoid exposure to chemicals, additives, pesticides, herbicides, and all other potentially toxic substances.

By making these dietary changes, it would no longer be necessary to measure portions of Larry's food. He could eat as much of the recommended foods as he wanted, and large fluctuations in blood sugar would be prevented because he would be eating foods with minimal tendency to raise the blood sugar. Regular exercise, along with B vitamins, magnesium, lipoic acid, and other nutritional supplements would further lower the necessary dose of insulin by allowing for even better blood-sugar control. Supplements could also protect body tissues from the damage caused by high blood sugars.

But it had taken Larry's parents two years to come to grips with caring for his illness, and they did not especially want to trade their hard-fought status for something unknown. They probably would never have sought a consultation with me had it not been for Larry's grandmother, a devotee of natural medicine. Though the parents thought they might learn something new, they were not prepared for something so different.

Our suggestions for Joanne's new diet met with similar resistance. When she came to our clinic for a nutritional consultation, Joanne had been eating a very large amount of refined carbohydrates like toast, cold cereal, waffles, honey, pasta, french fries, cookies, and popcorn. Like other children who regularly ate processed foods and fast foods, Joanne had developed a strong dependence on salt. I explained that so much salt in her diet was particularly dangerous for diabetics because it put them at risk of getting cardiovascular disease. I recommended that she eat more whole foods that didn't contain excess salt.

After her consultation, Joanne cried. She was upset about all the foods she would no longer be allowed to eat, especially Honey Nut Cheerios. She thought it was her own fault that she was overweight.

Major dietary changes like these that are required to successfully manage diabetes are hard adjustments for a family to make. But accepting the new dietary regimen becomes easier once everyone understands that these changes help to maintain diabetic control and the new plan is introduced slowly enough to gain the child's cooperation. What's important is coming to the realization that change can be successful without seeming overwhelming.

Changing the Family Dynamic

Still other problems occur when family members perceive the new diet as a threat to their own happiness. For example, Larry's father wasn't prepared to make lifestyle alterations to his own diet so that the entire family would be in sync with the new nutritional guidelines. Because he was unwilling to give up favorite foods like bacon, lunch meats, french fries, and soft drinks, his wife wound up cooking one meal for Larry and another for the rest of the family. When Larry saw what his father was eating, he felt deprived and angry, as well as less willing to stay away from the foods that would make his diabetes worse.

In time, most family members come to understand that changes made to benefit a diabetic child also benefit them. The recommended new diet is healthier for everyone. Eliminating saturated fats and trans fats, sugar, white bread, candy, and fast foods can save everyone trouble down the road. Children will be spared obesity, fatigue, allergies, skin rashes, and ultimate confrontation by the terrible trio of high blood pressure, heart disease, and adult-onset diabetes.

Childhood diabetes is a disease that affects the whole family. For the necessary changes to be made, group understanding and agreement are essential. When this is accomplished, diabetic children don't feel that they are imposing their illness on the rest of the family. Healing the diabetic child can be a healing process for everyone.

If Dad needs a jelly-filled doughnut, Tommy a milkshake, and Ellie a double order of fries with ketchup, they should fulfill themselves away from the home so that a diabetic child won't feel alienated by their choices. The recognition of being wanted and protected gives a child the strength to persevere through all the adjustments necessary to establish health. It's painful to watch the teasing and ostracism that kids suffer because they're different from their peers, and the loneliness and apathy they feel when they suspect that their illness has made them a burden to their families.

When everyone contributes to the effort, a victory for the child becomes a victory for the family. In time, the necessary changes become easier. Each family member becomes educated in nutrition, learning how to shop and even how to cook. The entire family also gains the health benefits gained by the diabetic child. Giving up doughnuts, milkshakes, and greasy fries will be good for Dad, Tommy, and Ellie!

Involving Your Child in Diabetes Management

Children who get diabetes can become fatalistic and feel that all is lost, no matter what they do. They may be angry, resenting that they have a problem they didn't cause. Family difficulties and new financial obligations can add to the stress caused by having diabetes.

It is paramount that parents not emphasize the complications of diabetes or enforce compliance without the child's understanding and agreement. It is the child, not the parents, who will ultimately achieve mastery over the condition. This will be an enormous victory for the child.

From the beginning, children should be involved in all aspects of treatment. They need to be educated, in words appropriate for their age and understanding, with pictures, definitions, and examples. Parents should remember that absolute observation of the regimen is not essential, especially in the beginning. Eating an ice cream is not going to require hospitalization, nor will missing a single dose of insulin. Changes in diet, nutritional supplements, and exercise need to be introduced gradually. Children should slowly assume responsibility for the daily tasks affecting their care by helping with shopping and food preparation. They should keep their own record of blood-sugar measurements. These activities can be organized as games, with points awarded as new tasks are completed and information gained. The points can be redeemed as privileges, trips, or games. To enhance morale, each little victory can be added to the others.

My crucial, inviolable rule, which I repeat many times over, is "Don't let diabetes build a wall between you and your child, and your child and the world." Faced with learning to cope with a difficult lifelong illness, it's essential that a child feel loved and supported. To make a child feel ashamed or in any way to blame for the illness can cause anger, resentment, and an unwillingness to cooperate in finding solutions.

Considering Home Schooling

If your child is not doing well because of this illness or an unsatisfactory situation at school, you may want to consider temporarily schooling her at home. This may help her to get more rest, eat better, and avoid distraction in a classroom that demands too much or offers too little. A child who has been diagnosed with diabetes may require more attention than a teacher can provide in a classroom of thirty children.

Home schooling can allow for nutritional controls not possible in school. It can also open many doors to parents who recognize that children's needs are not always met in a regular school. It opens doors for greater creativity. You can adjust the pace of teaching to match your child's ability to absorb information. You can handle confusion, because there's time enough to do so. You can provide more in-depth tutoring and concentrate more on your child's interests.

For those who worry whether their home-schooled children will find it difficult to adjust to regular school once they return, studies have shown that home-schooled children score as well or better on standardized tests as children in regular schools, regardless of how the parents were educated.

Some believe that home-schooled children can be deprived of social diversity and experience. My wife and I found the opposite to be true of our children. Home-schooled children can have very rich social lives. Children and parents can join groups formed especially for home schoolers. For suggestions and legal advice on the Internet, search the net under *www.homeschool.com.*

IT TAKES A FAMILY

In helping one child, the family redefines itself, and its members reaffirm their common strength and values. When complacency and self-interest are put aside, a health crisis can become a rallying point. Family members who strive for a common goal reinforce their own worth and the family's integrity.

Demystifying Diabetes Management

The goal in my practice is to demystify the ordeal of caring for a diabetic child by giving the family an easy-to-understand nutritional program designed to minimize the child's need for insulin and to blunt the high and low fluctuations of blood sugar. We prescribe a new diet and a variety of vitamins and supplements that not only reduce the need for insulin, but help to prevent the organ damage that diabetes causes. The program described in this book includes four basic steps:

1. Appropriate food choices: choosing foods with a low glycemic index (low simple sugars) and high nutrient density, avoiding refined foods and foods with additives and preservatives.
2. Optimal intake of nutritional supplements: this includes vitamins, minerals, essential fatty acids, and antioxidants.
3. A regular exercise program: to improve blood-sugar control, help maintain an ideal weight, and reduce cardiovascular risk.
4. Weight control: this must be a priority since Type 2 diabetes directly correlates with excess weight and the complications of Type 1 diabetes are aggravated by obesity.

These steps may seem simple and obvious, but diabetic children and their parents are often kept in the dark. Traditional diabetic care offers almost total emphasis on blood-sugar control using insulin and other medication, with poor dietary guidance and rare emphasis on nutritional support. In fact, the foods that nutritionists recommend—as we saw in Larry's case—often cause the very complications that they are supposed to prevent. It is no wonder so many children and their parents become frustrated. They never learned a better way.

But this book goes beyond providing an effective program for the management of children with diabetes. You should read this book if you:

- Have a diabetic child and have been told to let her eat whatever she wants, and just give her enough insulin to keep her blood sugar down
- Have a diabetic child whose doctor has told you nothing about how vitamins and minerals prevent deficiencies and complications
- Have a family history of obesity

- Have a child who is overweight
- Are committed to setting up your child for a lifetime of good health
- Are determined to avoid the dangerous pretense that kids can safely eat anything
- Are willing to make changes in your own lifestyle to help your child better manage diabetes.

CHAPTER 3

The Great American Obesity Epidemic

The term "obesity" is tossed around a lot these days, particularly in connection to diabetes. The most common definition of obesity is a body weight that is 20 percent above the acceptable range for a given height. It is important to remember, however, that the incidence of diabetes and cardiovascular disease progressively increases as weight rises above ideal levels.

In the past 30 years, there has been a 67.2 percent increase in the number of Americans who are obese. The highest increase was found in the state of Georgia—a whopping 101.8 percent. Clearly, there is an epidemic of obesity that is spreading across the United States. It cuts across all ages, but those who will suffer most are today's children. These children will spend more years of their life obese than any other Americans in history. Just how this will play out is evident in the disconcerting rise of Type 2 diabetes in children. Furthermore, because obesity is so closely tied to insulin resistance, many overweight children, although non-diabetic, will develop diabetes if they remain obese in adulthood. Most obese children, in fact, remain obese in their adult lives.

Measuring Obesity

Obesity is informally defined as body weight far in excess of ideal. According to the National Heart, Lung, and Blood Institute, the precise definition of obesity is a body mass index (BMI) greater than 30. To calculate your BMI, use the following formula:

$$BMI = Weight\ in\ kilograms\ /\ Height\ (in\ meters)\ squared$$

An ideal BMI is 25. Individuals with a body mass index higher than 25 are overweight. Assume for example that a girl named Tina weighs 176 pounds (80 kilograms) and is 5 feet 3 inches (1.6 meters) tall. Therefore she has a BMI of 80/2.56 (1.6 squared), which totals 31. Tina's BMI of 31 is just over the borderline of obesity. If she lost a couple of pounds, she would be just under the borderline. Of course, Tina needs to drop safely beneath that borderline.

A BMI over 40 represents extreme obesity. If Tina gains 50 pounds (23 kilograms) more to reach a total weight of 226 pounds (103 kilograms), she would then have a BMI of over 40 percent, which is considered extremely obese.

An acceptable body mass index for a child is lower than it is for an adult. As children grow, the body mass index normally increases. Higher than average increases, however, indicate that the child is gaining too much weight.

The following two charts from the CDC (Centers for Disease Control) can be used to evaluate your child's BMI based on percentiles for his or her age. To use these charts, first find your child's age on the bottom horizontal line. Then, go up to the 50th percentile line—the heaviest line—which represents the average BMI for that age. By reading across either to the left or right, you can find the body mass index number that corresponds to the 50th percentile. For example, the BMI for a twelve-year-old girl at the 50th percentile is 18 kg/m^2. The BMI for a fourteen-year-old boy, at the 50th percentile is 19 kg/m^2.

The higher your child is, beyond the 50th percentile, the more overweight he or she is. Thus, a twelve-year-old girl with a body mass index of 27 is at the 97th percentile and is much too heavy. She needs to lose weight to reduce her body mass index to 18.

Over the last 20 years, the number of obese Americans has risen to nearly a quarter of the general population. Over half of Latin and African-American females are obese. Worst of all, a

CDC Growth Charts: United States

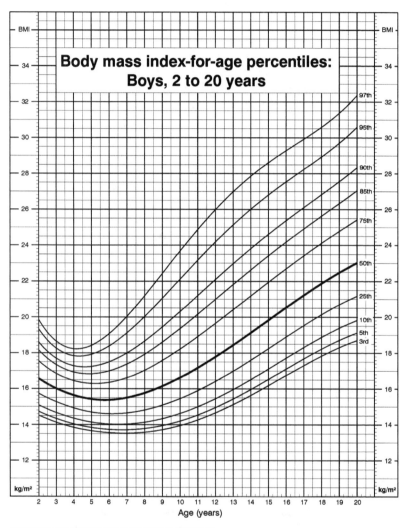

SOURCE: Developed by the National Center for Health Statistics in collaboration with
the National Center for Chronic Disease Prevention and Health Promotion (2000).

CDC Growth Charts: United States

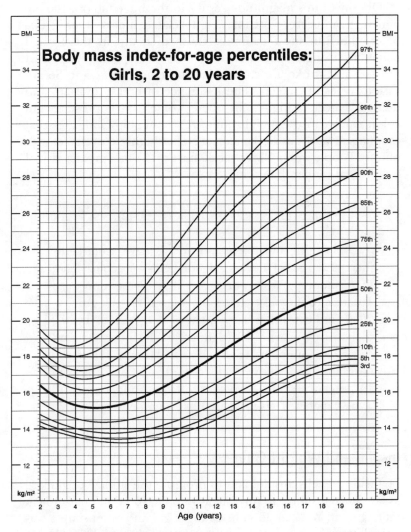

Body mass index-for-age percentiles:
Girls, 2 to 20 years

SOURCE: Developed by the National Center for Health Statistics in collaboration with
the National Center for Chronic Disease Prevention and Health Promotion (2000).

third of school-age children are obese. America is clearly losing the war against fat.

Obesity of this magnitude results in the huge tab of $100 billion in health-care costs for weight-related illness. Type 2 diabetes, the fifth most common cause of death in the United States, is strongly associated with obesity. Hypertension, heart disease, and stroke are closely tied to being overweight. So are various types of cancers. The incidence of breast, ovarian, and uterine cancer is highest in obese women, as is prostate and colon cancer in overweight men. A recent study indicates that esophageal and gastric cancer are also highly correlated with obesity. People with a BMI over 30 have a 16 times greater risk of esophageal cancer than thin people.

OBESITY INCREASES RISK OF DIABETES

Overweight and obese individuals have a markedly increased risk of developing diabetes. A report from the National Task Force on the Prevention and Treatment of Obesity (*Arch Intern Med*, Vol 160, Apr 10, 2000) indicates that 67 percent of people with Type 2 diabetes are overweight (defined as a BMI over 27) and 46 percent are obese (defined as a BMI over 30). In the past ten years, obesity has increased by 50 percent from 14 percent to over 22 percent of the population, and Type 2 diabetes has increased by 25 percent.

Insulin and Weight Gain

Inside fat cells, insulin acts to promote the storage of glucose as fat. Since insulin can turn sugar into fat, you don't have to eat fat to get fat! You can do so by eating sugar and other simple carbohydrates in excessive amounts. Foods that are quickly absorbed by the body, such as bread, fruit juice, and potatoes, raise your blood-sugar level rapidly and cause more insulin to be released. This insulin causes more storage of fat and a greater production of triglycerides (which along with cholesterol is one of the two major fats in blood). For reasons that are unclear, your appetite also increases, and you gain weight. Insulin itself has been identified as an independent risk factor for hardening of the arteries (arteriosclerosis.) Therefore, the more insulin you make, the greater your chances are for getting heart disease.

Other weighty factors

If your parents are obese, your chances of developing a weight problem are higher, both because of genetic predisposition and because of the eating patterns learned from them. Of course the odds can be reversed in your favor if you start eating a healthy, low-fat, high-fiber diet and exercising conscientiously.

Other environmental factors like the estrogen in hormone replacement therapy also can put on the pounds. Stress, too, can be a culprit, especially if you're an "eater" who heads for the refrigerator for comfort foods. Smokers who kick the habit often have to battle weight gain until they find a new way to cope with tension.

POSSIBLE LINK BETWEEN HOSTILITY, FAT, AND TYPE 2 DIABETES

A laboratory study at Arizona State University and an ongoing population study at Brown University found that hostile individuals put themselves at risk for coronary heart disease and Type 2 diabetes by having a cynical and mistrustful attitude. The results of the studies, which appeared in the January/February 2000 issue of *Psychosomatic Medicine,* found that hostility caused weight gain and increased blood pressure. Moreover, these hostile people had an exaggerated amount of body fat in the abdominal area, which can lead to insulin resistance and Type 2 diabetes. The researchers found that hostility leads to excess activation of certain stress hormones, in particular, cortisol, which causes body fat to be redistributed into the abdominal area, which in turn triggers problems with cholesterol, blood pressure, and insulin resistance.

> According to Raymond Niaura, lead author of the Brown study, "Somebody with a lot of abdominal body fat has stored fat (close to) the liver, which starts a chain reaction of increased cholesterol, blood pressure, and causes the insulin to be unable to do the job it's supposed to do." (*Wired News*, February 1, 2000)

Genetics Not Always Destiny

Each person possesses genetic uniqueness and biochemical individuality. Our genes, provided by our parents, establish our basic physical characteristics and our particular biochemical responses to stimuli in our environment. As a result, no two people look entirely the same, act the same, or react the same to experiences.

For example, after two people have eaten exactly the same food in the same amount, they will have different levels of blood sugar, cholesterol, hemoglobin, plasma protein, and thyroid hormone. Similarly, after two people take the same dose of aspirin, they have different blood-aspirin levels. The same applies to the metabolism of alcohol. After two people drink the same amount of vodka, one drives home safely and the other is arrested for drunken driving. Of two people equally exposed to HIV, one becomes infected and the other doesn't. When all other things are equal, differences in individual biochemistry make each one of us absolutely unique.

But our responses to different stimuli are not carved in genetic stone. Depending on how we modify our lifestyle, our biochemical makeup can change. For example, a patient of mine named Janice took eight Tylenol tablets a day for many years for her arthritis pain. Although Tylenol can damage the liver, Janice suffered no liver problems because her body could break down Tylenol into other, less harmful substances. When her husband died, and she started to drink heavily, her liver could not withstand the combined toxic onslaught of Tylenol plus alcohol. As a result, Janice developed liver failure and died. Her biochemical mechanisms served her well on one level, but couldn't cope when an additional toxic stress was added.

No matter how healthy or strong we are, any of us can be biochemically damaged to a point where sickness intervenes. The damage may come from a drug like Tylenol, a toxic food, such as alcohol, or a poison, such as a pesticide. In children with gluten sensitivity, eating substances like wheat products (which most people consider benign) can also trigger illnesses.

Groups of people with genetic similarities can have an increased risk for a particular disease. For example, Pima Indians living in Arizona have a 60 percent chance of developing Type 2 diabetes because of a genetic defect in the utilization of magnesium (which is important in the biochemical activity of insulin and in the utilization of glucose) that results in insulin resistance and diabetes. Weight gain seems to activate this defect. By comparison, Pima Indians who live in remote areas of Mexico and who lead more nomadic and physically demanding lives, are lean and diabetes free.

As you can see, genetics isn't necessarily destiny. The Pima Indians' genetic defect in magnesium utilization may be what predisposes them to develop diabetes, but it is not in itself sufficient to trigger the disease. Otherwise, the Pima Indians in Mexico, who also have this defect, would be getting diabetes. Their case is a good example of how a genetic defect sets up a susceptible state that allows diabetes to occur only when other factors, such as obesity and a sedentary lifestyle, intervene. Thus, by understanding the risks and modifying our behavior, we can prevent Type 2 diabetes.

The Energy Equation

No matter how much you eat or what you eat, you will lose weight if you burn up more calories than you take in. A formula for weight loss could be written like this: **Energy In < Energy Out:** Weight loss occurs when energy expenditure exceeds energy intake.

To keep trim, I give most of my attention to the **Energy In** part of the formula because it's easier to avoid calories than to burn them up. It takes an hour of extreme physical exertion to burn up 800 calories, but only minutes to devour high-calorie, high-fat foods. It can be awfully difficult to compensate for thousands of calories in ice cream and cake!

Television and Obesity

Once children were like whirling dervishes, inexhaustible internal combustion machines. They ran around all day long, getting into all kinds of trouble and turning a well-kept house into a distant memory. Today they watch television and play video games for an average of five or six hours a day. Watching television makes children fat, because the **Energy Out** part of the above equation greatly lessens. And don't forget, as one's weight increases, so does the risk of insulin resistance and diabetes.

A study titled "Reducing Children's Television Viewing to Prevent Obesity: A Randomized Controlled Trial" was published in the October 27, 1999, issue of the *Journal of the American Medical Association*. Its author, Dr. Thomas N. Robinson of the Stanford University School of Medicine, conducted a scientifically controlled experiment to measure exactly what differences in girth are to be found between kids who watch a lot of television and those who don't. He found that over seven months, television, videotape, and video-game use produced clinically significant changes in BMI, triceps skinfold thickness, waist circumference, and waist-to-hip ratio. In plain language, the video kids got fatter.

Overweight children are often unhappy and lack confidence. They don't perform well in sports and thus are even more likely to continue to sit around watching television and getting even more overweight.

If you want your kids to be healthy, fit, and intellectually challenged, television watching should be severely limited or even eliminated. Children need to use their energy in developing their physical and intellectual abilities to the fullest degree. To allow children to do otherwise invites a future of disappointment.

Food in the Fast Lane

It's only human to want to do what we like and to eat what we want without consequences. But life isn't like that. What we do and especially what we eat directly impacts our state of health and quality of life. We are what we eat. Poor eating habits almost invariably lead to poor health. As parents, it's our duty to act as good role models, eating healthy, nutritious food and teaching our kids to do the same.

It's wrong to set up children with destructive eating patterns to which they will become habituated. In my mind, it's a form of child abuse. Failing to teach kids about food is like failing to teach them to read and write—they will face life without the tools required for optimum success and survival. They will also become fair game for the relentless commercialism of fast-food profiteers, who offer toys with purchases of french fries and cheeseburgers.

It's not the genes we were born with as much as the food we eat that makes us obese and ups our risk of developing diabetes or undermines our control over the disease.

The chief culprit is a unique and insidious American invention—fast food. And it's darn near impossible to escape.

You encounter the message as you drive down the street with your kids in the car: Carl's Jr., Jack-in-the-Box, Burger King, Taco Bell, McDonald's, Denny's, Arby's, Wendy's, KFC, Del Taco, Roy Rogers, Baskin-Robbins, Ben & Jerry's, Häagen Dazs. The message is broadcast to your children in large, glaring signs: two miles to the next one. If you miss that one, there will soon be another.

The message even pays house calls. It enters your home through the television set, which subjects your children to endless propaganda.

To parents, the message is that you are tired, work too many hours, and are under too much stress. Fast food is easy. Each home has its own convenience store. Kids can go from box to box of cereal, crackers, nachos, and chips, washing it down with a sweet soft drink.

You can see the message in your local supermarket. Soft drinks extend perhaps 70 feet down one aisle. There are 68 varieties of sodas, five tiers high. There are 146 different snack foods, including potato chips, pretzels, corn chips, cheese puffs, tortilla chips, nachos, onion rings, and popcorn. There are 142 kinds of wheat wafers, wheat thins, crackers, popcorn cakes, and rice cakes. There are 172 kinds of cookies, 46 kinds of tarts and cereal bars, 160 kinds of candy. There are 136 varieties of cereal. Row upon row of sugar and refined grains, heavily salted, full of additives, preservatives, and colorings. For example, one cereal contains 15 grams of sugar per cup and five different food dyes. Fast food chains vie for the right to serve cheeseburgers, french fries, hot dogs, and pizza in school lunchrooms. Should anyone be surprised that kids are overweight? Soft drinks are everywhere, especially at home. You can sometimes buy Coca-Cola cheaper than filtered water. When I last visited Children's Hospital of Pennsylvania, one of the foremost medical institutions in the country, there was only one public restaurant on the ground floor—McDonald's!

The food served in hospitals to both children and adults is greasy, gravy-laden, and loaded with starch. Desserts tend to be chocolate cake and ice cream. Patients hospitalized with heart attacks have complained to me about being served bacon and eggs, rolls and butter, coffee with cream. It's a memorable experience to see a man sitting in bed, with an IV in his arm, an oxygen cannula in his nostrils, electrodes connected to his chest, eating meat loaf with mashed potatoes and gravy with pasty cherry pie waiting for dessert.

Kids are conditioned early in life, by their parents, schools, and television advertising, to eat foods that will lead them progressively toward obesity and diabetes. Commercials for fast-food restaurants craftily offer specials on Star Wars toys to kids who need only come in and order the special of the day to be awarded their prize.

A sure way to get children to eat something is to have it in the house. An even surer way is to set an example by eating it in front of them. Doughnuts, cakes, ice cream, cookies, pies, root beer, bread, croissants, bagels, french fries, sweet rolls, crackers, popcorn, pretzels, wheat thins, nachos, boxed cereals—the list is long. Eventually, children expect these foods to be available and resist eating healthier replacements. A struggle ensues, and the child usually wins.

When her parents brought her to my office for help in managing her weight problem, an obese 10-year-old cried inconsolably after the nutritionist told her that some favorite snacks would need to be eliminated. Her mother, who was also overweight, shook her head at the nutritionist's advice. The girl never returned for follow-up.

Without parental support in making lifestyle changes, the outlook for altering childhood obesity is not good. The parent needs to understand and accept the need for change, and the locus for change is in the home. This is where children learn the eating habits that they will have for the rest of their lives. That is why a child needs strong parental support and guidance in making the right food choices.

Children are brilliant students. They can precisely duplicate the attitudes and behaviors they see in their parents, whether or not their parents desire it. Their standard is the example set for them by their parents. If the behavior is pleasurable or addictive, it's especially likely to take hold.

There's a big difference, of course, between an addiction to drugs and a habit of eating bad foods. It's important, however, to recognize that habits acquired early in life and continually reinforced at home, in school, and during social events can be very hard to break. Overweight children often become overweight adults and, as adults, maintain the same eating habits they had as children.

In the name of efficiency and instant gratification, we are creating a society of people addicted to bad foods. We are setting our children up to be fast-food junkies. The current escalation of obesity and diabetes is a result of this. And obesity can be deadly.

Obesity and Cancer

Obese people get more cancer. They get more colon and rectal cancer, postmenopausal breast cancer, uterine cancer, and kidney cancer. While the reasons for this are multiple, some of the following factors are often involved:

- Obese people tend to eat a lot of processed fast foods and snacks, sugar, and simple carbohydrates. Fast foods contain saturated fats, which are implicated in the development of colon and prostate cancer.
- Obese people usually have a low intake of natural foods, like fresh vegetables, that contain cancer-preventing phytochemicals. The cruciferous or cabbage family is particularly rich in anti-cancer nutrients. More fruits and vegetables and less meat in the diet reduce the level of beta glucuronidase,

an enzyme produced by colonic bacteria that stimulates carcinogenesis.

- Obese people have higher levels of free sex hormones (i.e., not bound to protein and therefore biologically active) such as free estrogen and free testosterone, which are uniquely able to promote the growth of hormone-sensitive cancers, such as in the breast, uterus, and prostate.
- Obese people don't eat soy protein very often. Soy products, especially soybeans, contain isoflavones, which protect against breast, endometrial, ovarian, prostate, and colon cancers, as well as lymphoma and leukemia. These isoflavones—called genistein, daidzein, and glycitein—possess hormone-blocking effects. They are now available in soy-protein powders at most health food stores. Since soy is high in protein and vegetable fats and lacks sugar, it helps to control blood sugar and weight.
- Overweight people often don't get enough lignins, which are other plant compounds with cancer-fighting powers. Lignins are found in soy products and whole grains, but not in simple carbohydrates.

A diet that protects you from obesity also protects you from diabetes, cancer, and cardiovascular disease. The right diet and lifestyle make a big difference in controlling diabetes and maintaining good health.

FOR YOUTHS, "VEGETABLE" OF CHOICE IS FRIED POTATO

A *New York Times* article in September 1999 quoted a biomedical researcher at Louisiana State University who found that more than a quarter of the vegetables eaten by children are potato chips and French fries. For teenagers, these foods comprise one third of the total vegetables they eat.

Aren't French Fries Vegetables?

The staple of the American diet is the potato, consumed in far larger amounts than any other vegetable. It represents more than a third of the average American's total vegetable intake. That might be acceptable if potatoes were eaten as they're grown, with the jacket on, some seasoning, and a minimum of added fat. Instead, potatoes are usually eaten in the form of French fries, which makes them nutritionally very different from the parent vegetable, as the following table illustrates:

	Calories	Water	Fat	Saturated fats	Sodium
Baked potato with skin (7 ounces)	220	144 gm	0.2 gm	0.1 gm	16 mg
French fries (7 ounces)	632	76 gm	33.2 gm	10 gm	432 mg

Changing a potato into French fries removes half the water and adds enormous quantities of fat and salt. The potatoes are fried in partially hydrogenated vegetable oil. They used to be fried in lard.

Half the calories in French fries are derived from saturated fats or trans-fatty acids used in the cooking process. When the fries taste bad, it's usually the result of being cooked in rancid oil. Rancid oils are oxidized and add to problems with atherosclerosis.

A baked potato, on the other hand, contains almost no fat. Its calories are derived almost completely from starch, plus three grams of protein. The more foods are processed, the more likely they are to be depleted of vitamins and minerals and to contain undesirable additives.

It is important to emphasize that diabetics, because of the damage caused by elevated blood sugars, are at increased risk of vascular complications. It is also important to realize that vascular disease is simultaneously worsened by multiple risk factors acting in concert. Foods high in salt—such as French fries—contribute to high blood pressure, which adds to the vascular disease that occurs in diabetics, thus causing more vascular disease. Foods such as French fries also raise cholesterol and thus add another risk factor. Finally, foods such as French fries contribute to obesity, still another risk factor. Thus, when a natural food such as a potato is processed into French fries, it very well may promote vascular and heart disease in a diabetic by raising weight, blood pressure, and cholesterol, all at the same time.

CHAPTER 4

High-Risk Foods

The Trouble with Cow's Milk

What I'm about to say flies in the face of tradition and convention. Don't feed any child under age 2 cow's milk. It causes highly allergenic reactions, increasing respiratory problems and skin rashes. I've seen ear infections, chronic stuffy noses, sinusitis, and puffy eyes cured when children stopped drinking milk. It's even suggested, but not proven, that consuming dairy products increases the risk of developing Type 1 diabetes.

Why? The cows that produce milk are fed antibiotics to prevent infection and growth hormone to increase milk production. Both are present in milk. The food cows eat contains pesticides. They are also present in milk.

Milk is pasteurized to kill bacteria. It is homogenized to break the milk fat into smaller particles that will remain in suspension and not rise to the top. These smaller fat globules increase the rate of arteriosclerosis.

Compared to human milk, cow's milk is high in sticky, saturated fats and low in essential fatty acids. Many people can't digest lactose, the sugar in milk, and develop gas, bloating, and diarrhea when they drink milk.

Dairy products in general are deficient in essential fatty acids, iron, magnesium, and zinc. They increase cholesterol and triglyceride levels. They also increase blood clotting.

My wife nursed our son until he was two years old. Later, when he began drinking cow's milk, he became easily fatigued, with a stuffy nose, dark circles under his eyes, and excessive gas and bloating. Three days after he stopped drinking cow's milk, these symptoms disappeared. The sugar contained in milk is lactose. Many people lack the enzyme lactase, which is necessary for digesting milk. They develop gas, bloating, abdominal cramps, and diarrhea from milk and milk products. I have watched children with abdominal cramps and a failure to thrive improve rapidly when milk was discontinued.

Evidence of milk's health risks

A study of children with chronic sleeping problems revealed that one in nine got better when milk was removed from the diet. Symptoms recurred when drinking milk was resumed (Source: *Feeding Your Child for Lifelong Health* by Susan Roberts and Melvin Heyman).

Several studies have suggested cow's milk as a possible trigger of Type 1 diabetes ("Cow Milk and Insulin Dependent Diabetes Mellitus: Is There a Relationship?", *Am. J. Clin. Nutr.,* 1990, pp. 489–491; "A Bovine Albumin Peptide as a Possible Trigger of Insulin-Dependent Diabetes Mellitus," *New Eng. J. Med.* 1992, pp. 302–307). Infants given cow's milk may develop gastrointestinal bleeding and iron-deficiency anemia ("Cow Milk Feeding in Infancy: Further Observations on Blood Loss from the Gastrointestinal Tract," *J. Pediat.,* 1990, pp. 11–18).

Persistent advertising has touted milk as an indispensable source of calcium. Yet research has shown little effect of dairy products on osteoporosis ("Dietary Calcium Intake and Rates on Bone Loss in Women," *J. Clin. Invest.* 1987, pp. 1979–1982). In fact, high-protein foods, including milk, contribute to calcium loss through the kidneys. Countries with the highest per capita intake of milk—Holland, Denmark, and Sweden—also have the highest incidence of hip fractures (*Milk: The Deadly Poison* by Robert Cohen). The calcium in kale is more easily absorbed than the calcium in milk ("Calcium Absorption from Kale," *Am. Coll. Nutr.,* 1990, pp.656–657).

Cow's milk has been implicated as a cause of sudden infant death ("Cow Milk Allergies and Sudden Infant Death," *The Lan-*

cet, vol. 344, Nov. 5, 1994). There is also a suggested relationship between cow's milk ingestion and the development of cataracts ("Lactose and Cataract in Humans: A Review," *J. Amer. Coll. Nutr.,* 1991, pp. 79–86) and ovarian cancer ("Galactose Consumption and Metabolism in Relation to the Risk of Ovarian Cancer," *The Lancet,* 1989, pp. 66–71).

Alternatives to cow's milk

After reading the above, don't conclude that your children must go without milk altogether. There are several suitable substitutes for cow's milk, with mother's milk the clear winner for infants and children under 2 years old. Thirty years ago, in their excitement over the development of formula milk, experts maligned breast-feeding. Now all that has changed; pediatricians advocate breast feeding whenever possible.

Next to mother's milk, goat's milk is the best choice. Similar in composition to mother's milk, it is easier to digest than cow's milk. Soy milk is nutritionally excellent but should not be ingested by children under 18 months of age because of its allergenic tendencies. Rice milk is acceptable for healthy infants and children in small amounts, but should not be used by diabetics because of its high concentration of simple sugars.

Because they think only milk can provide the calcium necessary for bone growth, parents are often afraid to stop feeding their children cow's milk. That fear is no longer justified, as both rice and soy milk are now fortified with calcium.

Calcium can also be found in sesame seeds, almonds, soybeans, chickpeas, and beans as well as in many nutritional supplements. Children don't need cow's milk to grow.

If you provide cow's milk to your older children, try to obtain organic milk. It tastes much better and is free of pesticides, antibiotics, and hormones, including growth hormone. As with all other foods, organic is better.

America's Deadly High-Fat Diet

The American diet is high in fats, but not good fats. We don't eat enough fish, beans or lentils, or whole grains, which are the major sources of essential fatty acids (good fats). Our intake of omega-3 fatty acids is low, replaced by trans-fatty acids in fried foods, pastries, and snack foods, and by stearic, arachidic, and myristic saturated fatty acids in beef, lamb, pork, and dairy products. These fats make blood platelets hyperaggregable and red blood cells sticky. Red blood cells should flow separately within arteries. After a double cheeseburger and fries, you can look at a peripheral blood smear and see red cells lined up next to each other like a chorus line. I think it will be only a matter of time before research demonstrates increased rates of stroke and heart attack in customers leaving fast-food restaurants.

Another dangerous dietary fat, cholesterol, is not strictly a fat but a steroid. In the bloodstream, cholesterol is intimately bound to particles of fat and protein, with your level of cholesterol reflecting the amount of fat to which it is connected. Concern about cholesterol levels over the last 30 years has unfortunately given a bad name to all dietary fats. The Pritikin and Ornish programs for treating heart disease focus on very-low-fat diets, with less than 10 percent of calories coming from fats. These diets exclude fish, our major source of omega-3 fatty acids. They even exclude avocados because of their high oleic-acid content, which is also an ingredient of olive oil. Some individuals, especially prediabetics and diabetics, don't fare well on very-low-fat diets. Their triglycerides go up, their HDL, or good cholesterol, goes down, and their blood sugar rises, which can result in cardiac problems. A high intake of starches and simple carbohydrates, such as bread, pasta, and potatoes, is partly responsible, but so, too, is an excessive restriction of essential fatty acids.

Dietary Fats and Diabetes

Because diabetics are particularly susceptible to vascular disease, they need to be aware of how dietary fats can be supportive or damaging to blood vessels, depending on their structure. Vascular diseases do not develop in a month or a year, but over decades as the end result of incremental deposits of cholesterol and calcium in arterial walls, with coexistent inflammation. Eating high levels of undesirable dietary fats over a long period of time sets the stage for serious and life-threatening vascular complications, including heart attacks, strokes, and occlusion of the blood vessels to the legs.

Good fats, on the other hand, are protective and maintain the integrity of blood vessels. They counteract the damage produced by bad fats. (For a full discussion of these good fats, see chapter 6.) Good fats, such as omega-3 and omega-6 polyunsaturated fatty acids, are found in vegetables, grains, and fish. Bad fats are the saturated fats found in meat, fowl, and dairy products.

The picture gets more complicated when you realize that the body can produce fat from non-fat foods, such as sugars. Thus, by eating bread, you can increase the level of triglycerides, a form of fat that contributes to arteriosclerosis.

All children should be tested for the levels of cholesterol and triglycerides in their blood at an early age. Diabetic children should be tested on a yearly basis, since they are even more sensitive to the adverse effects of elevated lipids (fats). If your child's cholesterol is over 180 and triglycerides are over 100, there is an urgent need for a change in diet in order to prevent vascular disease later in life.

Terrible Trans-Fatty Acids

The introduction of trans-fatty acids to the American diet constitutes one of the great health frauds of modern times. Trans-fatty acids are formed by hydrogenation, the addition of hydrogen atoms to polyunsaturated fatty acids, such as vegetable oils. Hydrogenated fats or oils can be kept without getting rancid for much longer periods than unsaturated oils. In addition, hydrogenation makes fats solid at room temperature, improving their texture and spreadability.

Polyunsaturated fatty acids, such as fish oils and flaxseed oil, are fluid at room temperature. They can be poured. But they spoil quickly on exposure to light, air, or heat. Since total hydrogenation would make fat too hard, partial hydrogenation is used. Partially hydrogenated vegetable oils are present in almost all packaged foods. These oils are cheaper to make than butter. Advertising would have you believe they are safer. They are not.

Margarine contains trans-fatty acids ranging from 10 to 50

percent of total product weight; vegetable shortening about 20 percent by weight, and vegetable salad oil about 15 percent. Every day Americans eat, on average, 40 grams (8 teaspoons) of shortening and margarine containing about 10 grams (2 teaspoons) of trans-fatty acids.

A recent study by A. Ascherio and co-workers ("Trans Fatty Acids and Coronary Heart Disease," *New Eng. J. Med.*, June 24, 1999, pp. 1994–1998) underlines just how dangerous such eating patterns are to health. Their research indicates that trans-fatty acids have greater adverse effects on cholesterol levels than saturated fats. Fast foods loaded with trans-fatty acids need not contain this information on the label and can even be advertised as cholesterol-free and cooked in vegetable oil. While trans-fatty acids come from vegetable oils and contain no trace of cholesterol, they do affect cholesterol levels after they are metabolized. Because trans-fatty acids raise the level of LDL, or bad cholesterol, and reduce the level of HDL, or good cholesterol, they are considered the most dangerous of dietary fats.

In the study, Ascherio made the following observation: "When ingredients with no known nutritional benefit are added to foods, a low threshold for evidence of harm should be adopted, and it should be the responsibility of food manufacturers to show that their products are safe."

What does all this mean to you in caring for your diabetic child? For optimal health, avoid packaged foods containing partially hydrogenated oils. In fact, if you ever see the word "hydrogenated" on a list of ingredients, don't buy that food product. Keep in mind that trans-fatty acids are found in a lot of prepared foods, including fast foods, snacks foods such as chips and pretzels, and commercial bakery products made with margarine and vegetable shortening such as doughnuts, pies, and cookies.

THE ADVERSE HEALTH EFFECTS OF
TRANS-FATTY ACIDS

These are the most important effects on diabetics, as
they lead to accelerated arteriosclerosis:

- Increase insulin resistance
- Raise LDL, or bad cholesterol, levels
- Lower HDL, or good cholesterol, levels
- Increase triglyceride levels
- Interfere with essential fatty-acid metabolism
- Replace desirable fats in cell membranes, making
  the membranes stiff and dysfunctional
- Increase levels of lipoprotein A, a substance that pro-
  motes arteriosclerosis
- Impair immune function
- Decrease testosterone levels
- Interfere with pregnancy and cause low birth weight
- Reduce breast-milk production
- Adversely affect liver detoxification
- Associated with increased incidence of cancer

High-Protein Diet Problems

Type 2 diabetes is intimately associated with obesity, and the
rampant obesity in our society has promoted a frightening increase in diabetes. Thus, a diet that reliably reduces weight would
also reduce the incidence of Type 2 diabetes.

Americans are always in search of the Holy Grail of diets that
will promote rapid weight loss with a minimum of deprivation.
Like the high-protein diet. According to this diet, you can eat unlimited quantities of eggs, bacon, ham, sausage, liver, beef, steak,
salami, hot dogs, fish, chicken, emu, ostrich, cheese, beans, and
tofu. Animal and vegetable proteins are recommended equally.

A high protein intake does indeed suppress appetite, and
many people do lose weight on it. The theory behind such diets
is that high protein causes ketosis, an acidic state in the blood

that suppresses hunger. Although such diets have been effective in treating seizure disorders, especially in children, major problems are associated with their use:

- High-protein diets can cause nausea, headaches, and malaise (a general feeling of misery).
- After three or four weeks on such a diet, some people develop an uncontrollable craving for carbohydrates of all kinds and quickly regain weight lost.
- High-protein diets cause gout and worsen osteoporosis. The acid in protein is neutralized by alkali from bone, and calcium is lost in the urine. Vegetarians whose diets are usually low in protein and calcium have less osteoporosis than people who eat animal products.
- High-protein diets worsen kidney disease. Individuals with kidney trouble should restrict their protein intake.
- High-protein diets are low in fiber, a valuable source of nutrients. Fiber is metabolized in the intestine to form short-chain fatty acids, which feed and maintain the inner lining of the intestine. High-fiber diets are associated with lower rates of cancer.
- Animal protein alters the microbial population in the gut, establishing an environment that favors constipation, diverticulosis, and cancer.
- The incidence of colon and rectal cancer is increased in those who eat red meat. Folic acid that protects against colon cancer is found mainly in fruits and vegetables, not in meat.
- Animal products have a higher concentration of pesticides and herbicides than plants. The higher up the food chain you go, the more poison you find in your diet. Domestic animals are treated with hormones and antibiotics to increase their growth rate and viability. People who eat meat are also ingesting these substances. The impact these hormones and antibiotics have on health is as yet unknown.
- Meat diets are enormously wasteful of natural resources. Most of the grains grown in the United States are used to feed livestock, not people. It takes eight pounds of grain to obtain a pound of beef, and three pounds to obtain a

pound of chicken. Millions of tons of domestic animal wastes pollute rivers. The destruction of rain forests to make grazing lands is another of the many ecological consequences of raising livestock in huge numbers. The wholesale exploitation and slaughter of domestic animals by the billions are unnecessary, since no human body requires 20 servings of meat a week.

As harsh as this may sound, I don't intend to vilify meat eaters. I believe that most people, particularly children, can benefit from integrating animal products into a primarily vegetarian diet. But nobody needs a pound of meat a day. The solution to our problems with obesity, diabetes, and vascular disease will not be found in the butcher shop or in any rigid dietary ideology. People need variety in their foods.

Processed Carbohydrates and Sugar: A Shortcut to Diabetes

In February 1997, Dr. Jorge Salmeron and Harvard colleagues published the results of a six-year study that tracked the diets of 65,173 women 40 to 65 years old. The study, which appeared in the *Journal of the American Medical Association,* found that women who ate a low-fiber diet and drank a lot of soda became diabetic two and a half times more often than women who ate a healthier diet. The overwhelming message of the study was that women who ate a lot of sugar, pasta, white rice, and potatoes in order to cut down on fats in their food were harming more than helping themselves. Their diet of non-resistant starches (potatoes), processed carbohydrates (like white rice and pasta) and sugar (in soda) amounted to a shortcut to diabetes.

Starches are complex carbohydrates that comprise two groups—resistant and non-resistant starches. Resistant starches are slowly digested and metabolized and raise the blood sugar slowly after a meal. Thus, they create a small demand for insulin. They are found in foods like soybeans, lentils, certain grains such as millet, and some kinds of rice. Conversely, non-resistant starches such as found in potatoes, are rapidly digested and metabolized, and raise the blood sugar rapidly after a meal. Thus, they require greatly increased insulin production. In short, non-resistant starches impede blood-sugar control.

The above study was the first one to examine the effects of processed carbohydrates and sugar on a large number of people over a relatively extended period of time, and some of the results were startling. Although many people had recognized the dangers inherent in eating large amounts of sugar, until this research was published, few knew that some processed carbohydrates are even more harmful than sugar. The problem with such processed carbohydrates is that they cause the blood-sugar level to rise even more quickly than table sugar, triggering an even greater insulin response. Constant surges and high levels of blood sugar and insulin lead to obesity and insulin insensitivity, resulting in Type 2 diabetes. In the glycemic index discussed later in this book, various sugars and starches (all carbohydrates) are listed according to their ability to raise the blood-sugar level. Refined grains are the worst offenders. The next worst offenders are refined sugars and corn syrup. These simple carbohydrates are quickly absorbed by the body, triggering a rapid rise in blood sugar followed by a large secretion of insulin.

Whole Grains and Vegetables to the Rescue

Whole grains and vegetables contain complex carbohydrates that are more slowly absorbed by the body than simple sugars. As a result, they cause a more gradual rise in blood sugar, avoiding the need for a large secretion of insulin. Plant fiber is generally not absorbed by the body and thus causes no rise in either blood-sugar or insulin levels. In fact, fiber can help control your blood-sugar level.

There are several types of fiber, all from plants. Insoluble fiber (i.e., fiber that doesn't dissolve in water) includes cellulose, pectins, and lignins. They are found in green leafy vegetables and whole grains and seeds. They provide nutrition for the lining of the colon, increase the bulk and water content of stools, and have a laxative effect. They protect against cancer of the breast, uterus, bowel, and prostate. Soluble fiber, found in Jerusalem artichokes, leeks, garlic, and asparagus, support the growth of beneficial bacteria in the intestines. There are other varieties of fiber. But there is no fiber present in animal products. The average American adult ingests only 10 grams of fiber a day, one third of the recommended amount.

Enriched Flour: A Poor Choice

Enriched flour, the kind used in most commercially baked products, starts with the extensive milling of grain, which removes much of its fiber (bran and germ), essential fats, and vitamins and minerals like iron and the B vitamins thiamine, riboflavin, and niacin. While the flour produced may taste good, it's so devoid of nutrients that it actually causes nutritional deficiencies in people who eat diets that are high in baked white-flour products. The Enrichment Act of 1942, which required that lost nutrients be returned to white flour, was put in place to remedy this situation. However, the synthetic nutrients used to replace the lost natural nutrients don't remedy all the deficits created by the refinement process. This includes a loss of fiber, numerous vitamins and minerals such as magnesium and selenium, and essential fatty acids.

Because refined flour products lack enough fiber to slow down the body's absorption rate, they present a serious problem for diabetics. Converted to blood sugar very quickly, these cause a rapid rise in blood-sugar levels.

Sugar and Empty Calories

Our bodies were not designed to digest the huge amounts of sugar we now consume. In the early 19th century, each American ate about 12 pounds of sugar per year. In the early 20th century, that amount had risen to about 95 pounds. Since 1983, consumption of sugars and other caloric sweeteners has risen 28 percent. The average American woman has added 27 pounds of sugar, corn syrup, and other high-calorie sweeteners to her annual sugar intake. At the start of this new millennium, Americans are eating almost 165 pounds of sweeteners per person. And this amount continues to increase at an alarming rate.

In the average American diet, sugar is one of the main providers of empty calories. It contains no vitamins, minerals, phyto-chemicals, or fiber. The majority of these empty calories come from soft drinks, baked goods, and fruit-flavored drinks. Excess calories derived from sugar in food are stored as body fat in much the same way as excess calories from saturated fats. The end result is obesity, which sets the stage for Type 2 diabetes.

THE AMERICAN SUGAR RUSH

The average American's consumption of added sugar is skyrocketing, fueled by soda and snack food: 156 pounds of added sugar per person in 1999, up from 144 pounds in 1994, which in turn was up from 127 pounds in 1986.

According to federal surveys, the average teenager derives 19 percent of calories from added sugar, with the average boy consuming 34 teaspoons of added sugar daily and the average girl consuming 24 tea-spoons. Younger children, too, have diets far sweeter than desirable: 6- to 11-year-olds get 18 percent of their calories from added sugars.

For people with insulin resistance (between 10 and 25 percent of the population), a high-sugar diet forces their bodies to produce more than the normal amount of insulin, exceeding the ability of the pancreas to pro-duce enough insulin and resulting in diabetes. (Source: *The New York Times*, September 21, 1999.)

To cut down on your family's sugar intake, start by avoiding it in its visible and obvious forms. Don't add table sugar to food and drinks. Don't buy baked goods with sugar visibly sprinkled on top, and don't drink soda. The next step is to get in the habit of reading the lists of ingredients on food labels in order to elim-inate foods with added sugar. You will be surprised by how many there are.

Sugars Added to Foods

We consume enormous quantities of sugar. The average person ingests 20 teaspoons of sugar daily, and many individuals take in far more. One 12-ounce Coca-Cola contains 40 grams (8 teaspoons) of sugar. Its 155 calories are derived entirely from sugar. One graham cracker contains 8 grams of sugar. Two ounces of Frosted Mini-Wheats provide 10 grams of sugar.

In August 1999, thirty-nine health organizations petitioned the Food and Drug Administration to adopt the Agriculture Department's suggestion and issue guidelines advising Americans that 10 teaspoons of added sugar should be the maximum for someone eating a 2,000-calorie diet and maintaining a healthy weight. The health organizations also requested the FDA to require that food labels provide more information about added sugar.

In response, a National Soft Drink Association news release claimed that "the human body does not distinguish between added sugars and naturally occurring sugars," thereby suggesting it was pointless to distinguish between them on food labels.

Dr. Marion Nestle, chairwoman of the department of nutrition and food studies at New York University, says this claim "misses the point because fruit juices, for example, have phytochemicals, vitamins, minerals, and fiber, while added sugar provides empty calories."

I have treated many adult diabetics who were unaware of the huge amounts of hidden sugars in their foods, and many child diabetics whose parents did not realize how much sugar they were giving their children. Cold breakfast cereals and crackers are good examples of high-sugar foods that diabetics often consume instead of doughnuts or cake. Patients are often surprised to learn how much sugar their food contains.

IDENTIFYING HIDDEN SUGARS ON FOOD LABELS

Many food labels hide sugar content by calling it something else. The sugar most often added to foods is high-fructose corn syrup, which has very little fructose in it and acts in the body like any other undesirable sugar. It raises the blood sugar, makes it hard to control diabetes, contains no nutrients, and increases body fat. It also increases cavities.

In prepared foods, sugar can seem almost inescapable even where you would least expect it. To get around the problem, read the labels and pass up foods that have sugar listed as one of the first three ingredients, indicating it's one of the main ingredients.

To keep your sugar intake down, check labels for these substances:

Barbados sugar	Diastatic malt	Malt syrup
Barley malt	Ethyl maltol	Maltodextrin
Beet sugar	Fructose	Maltose
Brown sugar	Fruit juice	Mannitol
Cane-juice crystals	Fruit-juice concentrate	Molasses
Cane sugar	Glucose	Raw sugar
Caramel	Glucose solids	Refiner's syrup
Carob syrup	Golden sugar	Sorbitol
Corn-syrup solids	Golden syrup	Sorghum syrup
Date sugar	Grape sugar	Sucrose
Demerara sugar	High-fructose corn syrup	Sugar
Dextran	Honey	Turbinado sugar
Dextrose	Invert sugar	Yellow sugar
Diastase	Lactose	

SUGAR FACTS

- All sugars are simple carbohydrates quickly absorbed by the body with a tendency to elevate the blood sugar.
- Vegetables and whole grains contain complex carbohydrates that are more slowly absorbed by the body.
- Sugar is extracted from sugar beets or from cane in the form of raw sugar and molasses syrup. Raw sugar

can't be sold in the United States because of its impurities.

- Raw sugar is refined into white sugar, known as table sugar. It's almost pure sucrose.
- White sugar has no nutrients—only calories. The body has to use its own nutrient reserves to digest it. With high calories and low nutrients, sugar-rich foods can paradoxically cause obesity and malnutrition at the same time.
- Brown sugar usually consists simply of white sugar with a coating of molasses. It is no more nutritious than white sugar.
- Corn sweeteners, utilized increasingly in many foods, are sugars derived from cornstarch. They are no more nutritious than white or brown sugar.
- High-fructose corn syrup has been processed further with enzymes to increase its sweetness.
- Sucrose, dextrose, glucose, fructose, lactose, and maltose are all various forms of sugar. They are no more nutritious than other types of sugar.
- Honey is a naturally occurring kind of sugar. Although it has a slightly higher nutrient content, it's no better than other sugars.

Turning Kids into Sugar Junkies

Pharmaceutical companies are formulating children's medicines as candy, chewing gum, lollipops, and gumdrops. A child accustomed to soft drinks, ice cream, and the other multiple incarnations of refined sugar and artificial sweeteners falls easily into this new pharmacological calamity.

Apart from the fact that children are already overmedicated, we have the added danger of giving children an ever-increasing amount of sugar disguised as medicine! As sugar insinuates itself into children's tastes, it overwhelms other taste sensations. For example, young people accustomed to eating sugar are often repelled by the taste of vegetables. On the other hand, if kids are brought up on whole grains, vegetables, and fruits instead of sugar, they develop a taste for nutritious foods.

Habits and tastes developed early in life are maintained into adulthood. It is critical for diabetic children to learn good eating habits while they are young. Otherwise, they may have to resist the urge for sweets for the rest of their lives. When sweet foods are offered, they should be offered as a minor part of a broad nutritional program. Don't give your child a cookie or piece of cake after every meal, and certainly not a dish of antibiotic-laced ice cream. If you must include sweets, try making them with sweeteners such as xylitol or stevia, which are discussed later in this book.

Aspartame

Aspartame (Nutrasweet), a sweetener with poisonous effects, is now found in almost every food and drink with the word "diet" in front of its name. This includes all diet soft drinks plus thousands of other foods. Aspartame has a cloyingly sweet taste and an unpleasant chemical aftertaste. Because it contains no calories, some people think it's helpful in weight reduction. But several years ago, aspartame was responsible for more complaints to the FDA than any other so-called food.

Aspartame has been assigned responsibility for a variety of neurological problems, including headaches, dizziness, seizures, visual impairment, confusion, loss of concentration, numbness, tingling, ringing in the ears, gait disturbances, and weakness. I routinely ask patients who complain of headaches if they ingest Nutrasweet-containing food or drinks. Several have had prompt resolution of headaches after eliminating aspartame from their diet.

Aspartame is mainly composed of two proteins (amino acids), phenylalanine and aspartic acid. Both are considered excitotoxins, brain stimulants that cause neurologic damage. Phenylalanine increases seizure risk, blocks the production of serotonin, and has been associated with increased carbohydrate craving, PMS (premenstrual syndrome), insomnia, mood swings, behavior abnormalities, and depression. Aspartic acid has caused brain damage and genetic defects in experimental animals.

Methanol, another component of aspartame, causes blindness, headaches, lethargy, confusion, abdominal pain, and leg cramps. Additional toxins are released during the body's metabolism of aspartame: formaldehyde, formic acid, and diketopiperazine (DKP). DKP has caused brain tumors in animals, and formaldehyde is used as an embalming fluid.

Excitotoxins like aspartame have been implicated in the onset and progression of degenerative brain disorders including Alzheimer's disease, amyotrophic lateral sclerosis, Parkinson's disease, and Huntingdon's disease.

I don't allow any Nutrasweet-containing foods or drinks in my home, and I tell my children never to drink diet sodas. The potential risks are too great. It would actually be better to drink a regular soda, with its known and limited risks.

Although Nutrasweet has not been proven to definitely cause neurologic illness in humans, it has also not been proven to be safe. Despite thousands of reports of adverse reactions to Nutrasweet, the FDA continues to assert its safety. Of course, the FDA has also approved the marketing of many drugs that were later banned because of consumer sickness or death. Why subject your child to unnecessary risks? In the end, you alone bear responsibility for your child's health—not the government and certainly not the food manufacturers.

Sweet Solutions

Xylitol: a better sugar

As a sugar addict in college and medical school, I drank Cokes and chewed gum every day. One day, my dentist, who found 15 cavities in my teeth, gave me a rude awakening. Because sugar supports the growth of cavity-causing bacteria, I have suffered through many uncomfortable dental appointments since then.

As we've already discussed, sugar raises your blood-sugar level, making diabetes hard to control and turning to fat in your body. Yet Americans eat more sugar all the time, with both teens and adults consuming more than 150 pounds a year, nearly half a pound a day.

Ironically, the concerted effort to remove fat from our diet has resulted in the addition of even more sugar to make foods tasty. Sugar now seems to be in almost everything, making it very difficult to totally eliminate it from your diet. Replacing sugar with aspartame, currently the most popular sweetening substitute, is potentially toxic. In addition, it tastes bad and has an unpleasant aftertaste.

For those of us with a sweet tooth, there is a sugar substitute that both tastes good and is good for our health. Xylitol, a natural sugar found in plums, raspberries, and strawberries, is also found in birch trees, from which it is extracted for commercial use. With the same relative sweetness as sucrose, xylitol has just 2.6 calories per gram compared to 4 calories per gram in other sugars.

Because xylitol has a high fiber content, it is absorbed slowly by the body and causes only a slow and gradual rise in blood sugar. This makes xylitol good at soothing sugar cravings in diabetics without causing difficulty with blood-sugar control. I've found no change in the blood-sugar levels of diabetics who ate xylitol-containing protein bars. In a study, M. Georgieff and co-workers showed that replacement of sucrose by xylitol "results in significantly lower blood glucose levels and insulin requirements" ("Xylitol, an Energy Source for Intravenous Nutrition after Trauma," *Journal of Parenteral and Enteral Nutrition,* 1985, pp. 199–209).

Xylitol is extraordinary in other ways. Bacteria that flourish in other sugars don't like xylitol. Streptococcus mutans, which causes tooth decay, is inhibited by xylitol, as is streptococcus pneumoniae, which causes ear infections. In fact, zylitol chewing gum given to children halved their incidence of both tooth decay and ear infections.

I've added xylitol instead of table sugar to a number of recipes with excellent results and have included these in this book. When you use xylitol instead of table sugar, you'll find no adverse effects on blood-sugar control. However, taken in amounts greater than 40 grams, it may cause diarrhea. Xylitol costs much more than table sugar, so use it wisely.

Diane Lara, the nutritionist who wrote the recipes for this book, has created a protein bar using xylitol as a sweetener. Called Sugatrol RX™, it can be eaten as a snack without significant blood sugar elevations (see Resource Section).

Stevia

Stevia is a non-sugar herbal sweetener, 30 times sweeter than sugar. It contains no calories. Stevia comes from a small green plant found in Paraguay. As a sweetener it is available in tea bags, concentrate, tablets, powder, liquid extract, and ground leaf. Unlike artificial sweeteners, it is excellent for cooking and baking because it is not degraded by heat.

Because stevia is sweet but has no calories, it can satisfy the craving for sweets without making you gain weight. It inhibits the growth of bacteria and protects against tooth decay and gum disease. It may also lower blood sugar and blood pressure.

Stevia is completely safe. It is included in several recipes in this book. Use it in small amounts. A cup of sugar can be replaced with one-half teaspoon of stevia (see resource section for where to order stevia).

Dangers of Food Enhancers

Government agencies over the years have approved the use of chemicals added to foods to enhance production, preservation, or flavor. These chemicals were originally considered to be safe for human consumption when in fact they were not, as shown by subsequent events. Cocaine was once added to Coca-Cola. DDT was widely used for years as a universal insecticide for crops until it was found to be highly toxic to both humans and animals. Today, chlorine is added to drinking water, even though it is known to cause bladder cancer. Antibiotics are added to cattle feed, even though this promotes the growth of resistant bacteria that cause severe illness and death in humans (for instance, enteropathogenic E. coli in hamburger meat has caused numerous children to die of kidney failure).

Do not assume the intrinsic safety of food additives, preservatives, colorings, flavorings, hormones, and antibiotics. While everyone should avoid these toxic substances, diabetics need to be extra vigilant because they are more susceptible to the diseases that these chemicals can trigger. Thus, when a flavor enhancer such as monosodium glutamate (see next page) has a track record of causing adverse reactions in many people who ingest it, the reactions are even worse for diabetics.

MSG: The Unsavory Truth

Monosodium glutamate (MSG) is produced in the United States at the rate of 40,000 tons a year. It is added to a staggering variety of prepared foods, including fried chicken, frozen dinners, canned soups, sauces, sausages, seasoning salts, bouillon, meat tenderizers, matzoh balls, potato chips and most other snack foods, cured meats, lunch meats, and canned chili and stews. Fast-food restaurants use MSG in many of their products, such as Wendy's Crispy Chicken Nuggets, Jack-in-the-Box Breaded Onion Rings, Burger King Chicken Tenders, McDonald's Fish Filet, Arby's Fresh Pork Sausage, and Denny's Battered Cod.

MSG is often labeled on packages as hydrolyzed vegetable protein or as natural flavoring. It's also known as Accent, Ajinomoto, Zest, Subu, Chinese seasoning, Glutavene, Kombu extract, and Mei-jing.

What's frightening about MSG is that it often causes toxic reactions in many of the people who ingest it, often unknowingly. It's the cause of Chinese restaurant syndrome, a collection of symptoms including nausea, cramps, diarrhea, flushing, tingling, palpitations, headache, fatigue, drowsiness, and blurred vision. Other symptoms of MSG toxicity include depression, confusion, joint pains, wheezing, chest tightness, staggering, slurred speech, and dizziness.

Glutamate, found in MSG, is an amino acid that stimulates brain-cell activity. In rats, glutamate has been shown to cause brain-cell damage resulting in behavioral changes, seizures, and hormonal aberrations.

Both the developing brain and the aging brain are highly susceptible to toxins. MSG, though technically considered a food, may actually be a toxic drug. There is a high incidence of neurologic complications from drugs given to children, especially those passed in utero from mother to child. Older people react to drugs with confusion, memory loss, depression, loss of coordination, and an increase in falls and automobile accidents.

Twenty-five percent of people are allergic to MSG. Although its use has not been proven to cause long-term neurologic dysfunction in humans, neither has its safety been established.

Because its toxicity has been demonstrated in animals, it's foolish to expose children to it.

Of course, the food industry claims that MSG is harmless. But this is the same industry that has long shown a blatant disregard for human health in its pursuit of profits. Can its word be trusted in the case of MSG? I think not. I keep MSG out of my own home and advise my patients to avoid it as well. Unfortunately, MSG is hidden in so many foods that avoiding it entirely is almost impossible.

The Business of Food

The prominent American economist Milton Friedman wrote: "Few trends could so thoroughly undermine the very foundations of our free society as the acceptance by corporate officials of a social responsibility other than to make as much money for their stockholders as possible."

That's what drives American business for the most part. For example, toy, car, and gun manufacturers resist as too costly safety measures that most Americans want. For-profit hospital chains have been penalized for subjugating the quality of care to the bottom line.

It would be naive to assume that food manufacturers operate any differently. If they were primarily concerned with the health benefits of their products, half the items on supermarket shelves would not exist. In fact, food manufacturers are concerned almost totally with taste, convenience, and cost—factors that determine if a product will be successful. The effect of their foods on the consumer's health or life span is immaterial. But let's not be too hard on food manufacturers—they have to deal with the temptation of the trillion dollars a year that Americans spend on food.

The food industry's efforts to make money by promoting "health" has led to some colossal blunders. Margarine, one of these blunders, was first marketed decades ago, followed by other vegetable oils that remain solid at room temperature. The marketing strategy was to blame butter, lard, and coconut and palm oils for causing heart attacks and strokes, while claiming that margarine was safe. Many Americans switched to margarine, in all its varieties. Margarine turned out to be loaded with arteriosclerosis-promoting trans-fatty acids more dangerous than butter.

Although margarine has protected no one's health, it has made a lot of money. More recently, we have nonfat fats and spreadable oils made of mono- and diglycerides, which the ads say are good for you. At this point, we aren't even sure what these substances turn into after the human body has absorbed them.

Public concern about high cholesterol and obesity led to industry efforts to remove fat from commercial cakes, cookies, and other baked goods. In order to restore taste to the products, the manufacturers added sugar. A lot of sugar. Cholesterol levels have declined among Americans, but we are fatter than ever. No one bothered to inform the public that when the body absorbs excess sugar, it's converted to fat and stored. The American diet is now lower in fat, but higher in sugar and simple carbohydrates, and Americans are fatter than at any other time in our history. We have, as well, more cases of diabetes than at any other time in history.

The good news is that there is a growing number of food manufacturers who properly emphasize the nutritional value of their products. These companies cater to people whose foremost concern is health.

To provide the best nutrition for your diabetic child and your family, you should:

- Trust yourself, your own good judgment, and your strongly vested interest in your children's health.
- Become educated in basic nutritional principles and see that your children also get an understanding.
- Demand that your schools teach nutrition, beginning in the early grades.
- Insist that school cafeterias offer better food, preferably organic. If school officials say they can't afford it, ask for proof. Refuse to take no for an answer. Call your school board. Write your congressman. Positive changes are happening. They should happen also for your children, and they should happen now.

CHAPTER 5

A Safer Environment

A major purpose of this book is to emphasize the need to eliminate all damaging influences from your diabetic child's life. Ill health results from the combined insults of multiple negative factors. Poor diet, nutrient deficiencies, toxins, allergies, infections, and a host of other physical and emotional factors act together to damage a child's health. That's why it is important to examine the whole of your child's environment and to exclude all destructive elements.

Because we don't know for certain the cause of Type 1 diabetes, we cannot, with any certainty, blame it on dairy foods, dirty air, vaccinations, or antibiotics. However, we do know that toxic factors in a child's environment can cause a latent problem to develop into a full-blown illness. In other words, if several risk factors for an illness are already present, the disease process can be triggered by a seemingly unrelated outside agent.

Considering how vulnerable a diabetic child is to outside stress, it makes sense to do everything you can to protect him and the entire family from known toxins, polluted air and water, and unsafe foods.

Your Drinking Water

Because 60 percent of our body weight is water, it's fair to say that basically we're made of water. Water makes muscles strong, joints supple, and keeps all bodily systems in balance. Besides improving digestion, water lessens the risk of kidney stones, urinary tract infections, and actually reduces bladder cancer. It also helps keep weight down and energy level up. It is especially important for diabetics to drink sufficient amounts of water. When the blood sugar is elevated, it spills into the urine, causing an obligatory loss of water and other substances. This loss of water and nutrients, including vitamins and minerals, is called osmotic diuresis. Eventually, dehydration may occur, with weakness, cramps, and impairment of many body systems. Not only do diabetics need more liquids than other people, they also need to make extra efforts to ensure that the water they drink is free from toxins.

Children should drink a minimum of four glasses of water a day, and adults should drink six to eight glasses. In hot weather or during heavy exercise, even more water is required to maintain the body's internal balance. Otherwise, the body can become dehydrated, causing fatigue, light-headedness, and nausea.

While it's possible to live without food for a week or more, surviving that long without water is almost impossible. Fatigue sets in if there's as little as a 2 percent drop in the body's water balance. A 10 percent water deficit triggers major health problems. That's why it's essential for your children to drink a glass of water prior to intense physical activity, as well as two or more glasses afterward. Water breaks should be taken every ten minutes while working out. Since most kids have seen sports stars take water breaks on television, they won't need much persuading.

LIFELONG NEED FOR WATER

As the one ingredient that is absolutely essential for life, water:

- Makes up 83% of blood
- Makes up 75% of brain tissue
- Makes up 75% of muscles
- Makes up 22% of bones
- Regulates body temperature
- Conducts body waste through the kidneys

- Promotes intestinal absorption of nutrients from food
- Helps lungs absorb oxygen from air
- Assists in transporting oxygen and nutrients throughout the body
- Cushions organs against injury

Water promotes weight loss

No matter how balanced, tasty, and satisfying their meals, some people feel hungry all the time. Cravings cause them to pick at food constantly. Needless to say, they don't lose any weight.

What's surprising is that these hunger pangs may be thirst in disguise! In such cases, a glass of water will reduce feelings of hunger while a second glass taken a short while later can make them disappear completely. Try drinking a large glass of water before eating a meal and you will be surprised by how much sooner you will feel full.

Children should not feel deprived when they are given water instead of Dr. Pepper or a vanilla milk shake. They need to know that water is actually good for them. This, of course, leads to the question of whether the water from your kitchen tap is indeed safe for them to drink.

How pure is your drinking water?

According to the World Health Organization, 80 percent of illnesses around the globe could be eliminated if we all drank pure water. Pure water, however, is unavailable in many places. Even in developed countries, people are coming to realize that when they turn on a tap to fill a drinking glass, what they get depends very much on their location. In the United States, much of the water supply has been affected by sewage, pesticides, petrochemicals, and agricultural and industrial runoff.

The alarming truth is that our drinking water is getting more and more affected by pollution. Some of it is easy to see, but much is subtle. Five thousand new chemicals are introduced into operation each year. On an annual basis, manufacturing releases

18 billion pounds of chemicals and other pollutants into the atmosphere, soil, and groundwater. Together with agriculture, it uses more than 70,000 chemical compounds to produce products.

Given such statistics, it's hardly surprising that chemicals and organisms are being detected in water supplies that were absent only a few years ago. More than 700 of these chemicals have been detected in our drinking water, only 86 of which have clearly defined safety limits set by the federal government.

The good news is that water can be more easily purified than food or air. Whether the water in your kitchen tap is healthy to drink depends on how well the water in your city's pipes or country wells has been processed. You can't assume that water is pure just because it comes from a modern municipal system or from a rustic aquifer. As I've said before, where your children are concerned you need to play it safe. To ensure that their drinking water is healthy, purchase a good water filter, one that is able to remove all traces of chlorine, fluoride, microorganisms, and lead.

Purifying your drinking water

The safest water is filtered water. You can install small charcoal filters above or below the kitchen sink or attach them directly to the tap. Such filters remove chlorine, rust and other particular matter, and organic residues. The cost is one or two cents a gallon, much cheaper than buying bottled water.

A more elaborate water-purification system consists of a combination of reverse osmosis and activated carbon filters. In this system, the water is first passed through a sediment filter. Then, by reverse osmosis, the water is forced through a semipermeable membrane that filters out organic and inorganic particles. Before use, the water is stored in a pressurized tank. As it is being used, the water passes through activated carbon filters that eliminate any taste or odor.

If You Must Drink Tap Water

- Before you drink, let the water run for a short while in order to flush out the pipes.
- Don't use hot tap water to make tea. Hot water is more likely to have heavy metals and other chemicals dissolved in it than cold water.

Buying Pesticide-Free

To protect its citizens from pesticides, the U.S. government has outlawed the use of certain chemicals in farming. But the companies that produce these chemicals merely changed strategies by exporting them to other countries where their use is permitted. The irony is that the agricultural products grown in these countries are then imported into the United States to be eaten by Americans. Case in point: one border crossing with Mexico handles 700 trucks a day carrying fruits and vegetables. Thus, chlordane and other highly toxic chemicals that are illegal in this country may nonetheless have been used in growing many of the foods you purchase in U.S. grocery stores or restaurants.

Most pesticides are neurologic poisons. They can damage the nervous system as well as other systems in the body. DDT, for instance, was found to cause sterility and birth deformities in many animals. In the case of diabetics, who are prone to neuropathy (nerve damage), aggravating factors such as pesticides should be avoided.

The remedy is to buy organic produce whenever you can. It costs more but is safe, and the nutrient content of organically grown foods is much higher than conventionally grown produce. And remember to always wash your fruits and vegetables before eating them.

Dr. Andrew Weil's Dirty Dozen

Based on research by the Environmental Working Group, alternative medicine pioneer and author Dr. Andrew Weil picked the following eleven fruits and one vegetable as those most likely to contain high levels of pesticides. He recommended putting organic versions of these foods in your shopping cart:

Apples	Cherries	Pears
Apricots	Grapes, Chilean	Raspberries
Blackberries	Nectarines	Spinach
Cantaloupe, Mexican	Peaches	Strawberries

Are Genetically Engineered Foods Safe?

Thousands of products on supermarket shelves are now made with genetically modified organisms (GMOs). According to the *Wall Street Journal,* half of America's soybeans and a third of its corn are genetically altered. Genetically modified products are found in McDonald's hamburger buns, Betty Crocker cake mixes, Coca-Cola syrup, and many other commercial foods (see table below).

The biotech industry claims that no one has been harmed by eating GMO food. But doctors and scientists warn that there is not enough evidence to ensure that these foods are safe. They and an increasingly vocal segment of the population—particularly in Europe—have expressed concern about the long-term safety of products whose effects have not been researched. These people believe that in the absence of long-term studies, food manufacturers should not be treating people like guinea pigs. In the case of diabetics, it is always better to be prudent rather than sorry. Be vigilant about the foods you serve your diabetic child. Don't feed genetically engineered foods to them or anyone else in your family. As much as possible, try to buy organic food.

RECOGNIZING GENETICALLY ENGINEERED INGREDIENTS

In tests conducted in September 1999 by Genetic ID and *Consumer Reports* magazine, these brand-name processed foods were found to have genetically engineered ingredients:

Aunt Jemima Pancake Mix
Ball Park Franks
Betty Crocker BacOs Bacon Flavor Bits
Boca Burger Chef Max's Favorite
Bravos Tortilla Chips
Duncan Hines Cake Mix
Enfamil ProSobee Soy Formula

Frito-Lay Fritos Corn Chips
Gardenburger
General Mills Total Corn Flakes Cereal
Heinz 2 Baby Cereal
Jiffy Corn Muffin Mix
Kellogg's Corn Flakes
Light Life Gimme Lean

McDonald's McVeggie Burgers
Morning Star Farms Better'n Burgers
Morning Star Farms (GreenGiant) Harvest Burgers
Nabisco Snackwell's Granola Bars
Nestle Carnation Alsoy Infant Formula
Old El Paso Taco Shells
Ovaltine Malt Powdered Beverage Mix
Post Blueberry Morning Cereal
Quaker Chewy Granola Bars
Quaker Yellow Corn Meal

Quick Loaf Bread Mix
Similac Isomil Soy Formula
Ultra Slim Fast

The Lancet, a prestigious British medical journal, broke with tradition in its October 16, 1999, issue, in which it published the results of a study on genetically engineered potatoes. Researchers found that rats fed genetically altered potatoes developed the intestinal wall thickening typical of a reaction to a toxic substance. The toxin was thought to be lectin added genetically to the potato plant to help it resist insect attacks. While not conclusive proof, this is the first strong potential evidence that genetic engineering of food crops can be harmful to humans. At the very least, as the editor of *The Lancet* decided, this technology needs closer scrutiny.

Protect Your Kids Against Environmental Toxins

When my youngest son came home from school talking about a teacher who regularly sprayed ammonia on the desktops without concern for the effect it would have on youthful lungs, I started to think about the toxins in our environment to which our children are routinely exposed. Like the routine spraying of landscape for pesticides. Years ago, my neighbor's dog developed cataracts, hepatitis, and then leukemia, likely from the pesticides sprayed weekly on the lawn to keep it lush and green. This year after our back yard was fertilized, my own dog had two episodes of grand mal seizures. He had never had them before.

Our environment is so teeming with toxins, it's impossible to escape them all. Even the oceans and atmosphere are contaminated. Beaches are often closed because the water is contaminated with waste. According to newspaper reports, you have to go five miles out to sea from Key West at the tip of the Florida Keys to find seawater free of human sewage. From the hill I live on, I can see a layer of purple and brown smog enveloping the huge plain of Los Angeles and Orange County. The smog is denser in spring and summer, but never absent.

We may not be able to change how the world works as quickly as we'd like, but we can become more alert to environmental toxins like these and take steps to protect the young lives in our care:

- Some parents smoke cigarettes around their children, oblivious to the fact that passive smoking causes 3,000 cases of lung cancer a year.
- Food additives, colorings, and flavorings (such as MSG and aspartame) can cause some children to have headaches and difficulty concentrating.
- Antibiotics are given to children for countless cases of viral pharyngitis, sinusitis, and otitis, for which these drugs are known to be totally ineffective. These antibiotics can create yeast overgrowth, gastrointestinal problems, and dangerous antibiotic-resistant organisms. In addition, domestic animals treated with antibiotics carry resistant bacteria. When

they are slaughtered and fed to children, the children can contract overwhelming, sometimes fatal infections.

• Don't give your kids medications unless absolutely necessary. Ask their doctors to prescribe prescriptions only when they are really needed, and then for the briefest time required. Long courses of antibiotics often confer no advantage for cure and increase the risk of side effects.

• Buy organic foods whenever possible, even though they cost more.

• Try to use free range chicken and poultry which are raised on antibiotic and hormone-free feed (see resuorce section for where to purchase).

• Wash all fruits and vegetables.

• New rugs emit gases. Avoid them in favor of bare wooden floors.

• Try and use cotton bedding instead of synthetics.

• Use organic pesticides and cleansers.

• Check your home for radon.

• Don't use aluminum cookware. Aluminum is toxic to the brain.

• So is mercury. There's no reason for your children to have amalgam fillings in their teeth. Ceramic fillings look better and are safer. Take your children to the dentist regularly. Get their teeth straightened, if necessary.

• Give your children vitamin C to lessen the risk of lead toxicity.

• Investigate and treat your children's allergies. Allergies can lead to asthma and chronic gastrointestinal and skin conditions.

PART II

GETTING WELL

CHAPTER 6

Food as Medicine

Our bodies forgive us throughout our lives. They forgive our lack of sleep, our physical excesses, our use of makeup, body piercing and plastic surgery, excessive sun exposure, substance abuse, and bad food. *Up to a point.* At the point of illness, and preferably some time before, it is good to realize that our behavior can profoundly influence our health.

One of the most important realizations is that food can be medicine or it can be poison. What we put in our mouths and chew and swallow can make us sick or help us to become healthy. When you are ill, it becomes urgent to change your criteria for food selections because food can make you well. Conversely, the wrong food can make you sicker, or it can hasten your death. Meat is the wrong food for a person with gout, salted nuts for the person with leg swelling or high blood pressure, fried chicken for the person with heart disease.

No disease requires greater dietary restrictions than diabetes. There are many foods in our modern society that adversely impact diabetic care. They are the same foods that have made 50 percent of us overweight and raised the risk of heart disease.

When you read this chapter, try to think of food as medicine, of the importance of preparing food to heal your child in the same way you would choose her clothes to keep her warm. Good health becomes the concern above all others. In this way, you can open your mind to new ideas and attempt to tolerate things you would never have tolerated before.

Weight Control

Because weight control is so critical for diabetes management, it is important to create a diet plan that is both safe and works well over the long term. New diets arrive on the scene with predictable frequency. Though most of them work, their success generally lasts for a few weeks or a month or two. Then reality reasserts itself, and the dieters go back to eating what they've been craving for all those weeks and months of sacrifice. In the end they're no farther ahead than they were before. In fact, in addition to gaining back every ounce they lost, making up for their deprivation often results in additional pounds. Regardless of whether the new hot fad diet is predicated on a meal plan of rice, fruit, juice, cabbage, low fat, or high protein, unless it is comprehensive and sustaining, the diet will have a very short life and even more limited success.

To keep diabetic children slim and healthy, what's needed is a diet that can be maintained over the long term. That means one consisting of whole foods high in fiber and low in simple carbohydrates. Any item that comes wrapped or packaged is less likely to do them any good because such foods are frequently high in sugar, salt, fat, additives, and preservatives. The more children eat and become accustomed to whole foods, the more their taste for them will develop. Other foods will seem empty and unsatisfying. If they try to return to eating foods high in sugar, they will seem cloying and a little too sweet. The longer your children and you avoid sugar, the easier it will be for you all to continue avoiding it.

GOOD FOODS/BAD FOODS

Foods to Avoid	Foods to Choose
Fast foods	
COMMERCIAL cheeseburgers, hamburgers, french fries, hot dogs, fried chicken, chicken tenders, tacos, pizza	Homemade burgers, chicken, or turkey that are made from organic meat, chemical-free hot dogs, pizza
Junk foods and snack foods	
Pretzels, popcorn, corn chips, potato chips, cheese puffs, rice cakes, graham crackers, snack crackers, and similar items in bags with labels denoting "partially hydrogenated . . . oils"	Homemade snacks, raw sunflower and pumpkin seeds, almonds, walnuts, pecans, soy nuts, raw vegetables, apples, melon, pears, and other low glycemic-index fruits
Bakery items	
Donuts, cookies, pies, cakes, toaster pastry, twists, croissants—all loaded with trans-fatty acids, sugar, salt, and chemicals	Healthy homemade treats—cookies, muffins, cakes, and pies that are made from whole grain flour and no sugar or added fats
Soft drinks	
Regular or diet, all brands, colors, and flavors—loaded with sugar, high fructose corn syrup, or aspartame	Homemade lemonade or iced teas of all kinds, sweetened with stevia or xylitol; filtered or distilled water
Sugars	
White, brown, raw, fructose, high fructose corn syrup, honey, molasses, maple syrup, date sugar, artificial sweeteners	Stevia, xylitol, brown rice syrup (in small amounts)
Deli meats	
Hot dogs, bologna, ham, turkey, salami, pastrami (contain dyes and cancer-causing nitrites)	Natural meats
Oils	
Refined vegetable oils, margarine, and other artificial spreads	Extra virgin olive oil, organic coconut oil, or butter

Foods to Avoid	Foods to Choose
Mayonnaise	Homemade mayonnaise made with olive oil
Commercial salad dressings	Homemade salad dressings with olive oil
Nuts and seeds roasted in oils or purchased from bins (May be rancid)	Raw, unsalted nuts and seeds in sealed bags (store in refrigerator or freezer as nuts contain fats that can go rancid)
Commercial meats	Organic, free-range meat, chicken, turkey
Refined, processed grains (quick-cooking or instant) and refined flours	Whole, organic wheat and rye berries, oat groats, buckwheat, quinoa, teff, amaranth, Basmati rice, and brown rice
Chemicals, preservatives, artificial colors	None
Canned vegetables and fruits	Fresh or frozen organic fruits and vegetables
Canned beans and lentils	Home-cooked beans and lentils
Commercial eggs	Fertile, cage-free eggs, or omega-3-rich eggs
Fruit juices	Whole, organic fruits
Commercial breads	100% stone-ground whole wheat or whole rye, or sprouted-grain flourless bread
Regular potatoes	Small, red, new potatoes—in small amounts and mixed with other vegetables
Cold cereals (all of them)	Whole grain, long-cooking hot cereals
Commercial peanut butter (contains hydrogenated oils)	Organic, non-hydrogenated nut butters (peanut, almond, cashew, macadamia, tahini)
Sweets—candy, fruit leathers, gum, raisins and other dried fruits, ice cream, sherbet and sorbets	Homemade treats, ice cream made from plain yogurt (see recipes) using natural sweeteners (such as stevia or xylitol)
Cow's milk and cheeses	Goat's milk, soy milk, almond milk,

Foods to Avoid	Foods to Choose
	goat cheese (in small amounts), organic plain yogurt and goat yogurt
Ice cream, frozen yogurt, sorbets, sherberts, ice milk, popsicles, fudgsicles	Homemade frozen yogurts (see recipe), homemade popsicles made from Celestial Seasonings fruity iced teas.
Tap water	Filtered, distilled water, or bottled water

ALTERNATIVE SOURCES OF CALCIUM

Parents worry about calcium intake when milk is omitted. Milk provides 300 mg of calcium per 8-ounce serving. Here are some good substitutes.

Whole sesame seeds	1160 mg/100 gm (about 3 oz)
Kelp	1093 mg
Collard greens	250 mg
Kale leaves	249 mg
Almonds	234 mg
Soybeans, dried	226 mg
Brazil nuts	186 mg
Chickpeas, dried	150 mg
White beans, dried	144 mg
Pinto beans, dried	134 mg

The Truth About Eggs

Although eggs are rich in unsaturated fats, essential amino acids, folic acid, and other B vitamins, nutrition experts have been condemning eggs for years because of their high cholesterol content, which averages 213 milligrams per egg. The experts thought that eating eggs would result in higher cholesterol levels and increased rates of heart disease. However, a recent study revealed that in diabetics, the risks increased only for those eating more than one egg a day. There was no increase in the risk of heart disease or stroke in normal people eating any amount of eggs. (Source: "A Prospective Study of Egg Consumption and Risk of Cardiovascular Disease in Men and Women, *Journal of the American Medical Association,* April 21, 1999, pp. 1387–1394). Egg consumption may reduce health risks by raising the level of HDL cholesterol (the good kind) and reducing blood-sugar levels and insulin production. They can also provide welcome variety to a diabetic's diet. An egg, of course, is composed of whatever the hen eats. Hens fed flaxseed oil produce eggs tasting of flaxseed oil and are full of the omega-3 fatty acids found in flaxseed. Eggs that come from free-range hens, especially those fed sprouts, are the healthiest and best tasting, and have the least risk of containing salmonella.

SUPER EGGS

To create high-quality eggs, some farmers give hens special feeds. For example, Gold Circle Farms feeds hens algae containing large amounts of docosahexaenoic acid (DHA), the predominant unsaturated fat found in brain tissue, essential for optimal brain function. The resulting eggs contain 180 milligrams of DHA, 10 times more than regular eggs. Best of all, each egg costs less than a capsule of DHA—and it's a food! In one patient, eating DHA eggs lowered the cholesterol more than taking a cholesterol-lowering medication.

Eggs should be poached of soft-boiled so that the yolk remains semi-liquid when eaten. Some people prefer to separate the white from the yolk before cooking, adding the yolk at the end so that it remains liquid. This preserves the nutrients, including lecithin, which are otherwise damaged by heat. Cooking the yolk at a high temperature oxidizes the cholesterol and may promote atherosclerosis.

Try cooking a free-range egg next to a regular commercial egg. The shell of the free-range egg will be thicker and harder to crack. The yolk inside that egg will be densely viscid and a beautiful dark yellow. It will taste delicious, with an intrinsic hint of salt. The other shell, thin and fragile, will contain a yolk pale in color, limp and easily ruptured, tasteless and unsatisfying. Both are eggs, but very different in sensory qualities and nutrient value. The addition of eggs to your diet allows a big increase in variety of dishes.

Taking the Initiative

It takes knowledge, skill, and planning to escape the ever-present pitfalls of bad eating. American society has failed in this effort. Most parents do not learn or teach nutrition. Most schools don't teach nutrition. Medical schools have barely begun to teach it, and a study found medical students less interested in nutrition in their senior year than the year they entered medical school. You must take the initiative yourself.

That's what the parents of 2½-year-old Zach did.

Zach's Story

Because they had received no guidance about what foods to give their diabetic son after he was discharged from the hospital's intensive care unit, they came to see me. He was taking insulin twice a day, 2½ units of long-acting insulin in the morning, and 2½ units of combined long- and short-acting insulin before dinner. His parents had been told it didn't matter what he ate, just that he needed enough insulin to keep the blood sugar from rising too high.

Zach's diet was a diabetic disaster: numerous high-glycemic-index foods, including cold cereals, sodas, dried fruit, watermelon, bananas, raisins, graham crackers, bread, chips, and other snack foods. I explained to his parents that he needed to substitute low-glycemic-index foods in their place. I also prescribed the following nutritional supplements: biotin (a B vitamin that enhances insulin activity), 8 mg a day; chromium picolinate, 200 ucg a day; vanadium, 8 mg, three times a week; lipoic acid, 150 mg a day; and omega-3 fatty acids, 1 tablespoon a day. He also started on 5 mg a day of Leukomeal, a special nutrient that improves blood-sugar control. Leukomeal is derived from components of beneficial gut bacteria, including acidophilus and lactobacillus bulgaris. It increases the activity of insulin by suppressing the action of a white blood cell hormone called tumor necrosis factor alpha (see Resource Section).

A year later, Zach's blood sugar was in a desirable range, and there were no hypoglycemic reactions. Even though he wasn't yet 4 years old, he was testing his own blood-sugar level four times a day, with his parents' help. He was taking insulin twice a day, a combination of long- and short-acting insulin before breakfast and before dinner, a total of eight units a day. Although Zach did not enjoy the insulin needles, he didn't complain too much.

He was also doing gymnastics and swimming every week, and enjoyed them a lot.

Zach's parents changed their diet as well as their son's. They stopped drinking sodas and ate organic fruits and vegetables. It was not a difficult transition for them. Zach sometimes had popcorn and diet soda at school. He didn't have milk or regular cereals. He ate sprouted grain breads. He liked homemade yogurt with fruit.

As a result of these changes, there had been no interim visits to the hospital. Zach was active and healthy except for his diabetes. His parents felt much more secure in dealing with his condition.

Making changes like these isn't easy because learned patterns of eating are difficult to unlearn. In my own case, there were a lot of formidable forces, like the availability of fast food and the tastiness of "bad " food, that made it difficult to implement my good intentions. Nonetheless, over the last 10 years, I have unlearned my habits of drinking coffee and Cokes and eating fast foods and packaged snacks. Unfortunately, I have yet to unlearn other patterns of bad eating. It would have been far easier if I had never fallen into those patterns in the first place.

Only One Healthy Anti-Diabetes Diet

Keep in mind that in preventing and treating diabetes, there's only one healthy diet. This can have many variations but it must include the following: whole foods instead of processed foods,

foods high in fiber, low in saturated fats and trans fats, and low in refined carbohydrates. Eating this way is essential:

- To prevent your child from becoming overweight
- To help your obese or overweight child lose weight
- To best control your child's Type 1 diabetes
- To prevent your child from developing Type 2 diabetes
- To reverse your child's Type 2 diabetes
- To keep yourself, your spouse, other children, and grand-children healthy

Putting It All Together

Good nutrition, exercise and supplements are interrelated and absolutely crucial to the management of diabetes. Following the guidelines for one without including the others is a recipe for failure. To make sure the program works for your child, and that food is nutritious, easily digested, and turned into energy, follow these guidelines:

- Maintain food variety.
- Encourage kids to drink a lot of water—at least four glasses a day. But don't use water to wash down food instead of chewing it properly.
- Keep kids away from anything listing high-fructose corn syrup on the label.
- If you have diabetic teens, make sure they avoid alcohol.
- Young people, especially diabetics, should not drink coffee. It speeds the heart, irritates the stomach, and interferes with sleep. It doesn't do adults much good either.
- Add the recommended supplements to your diabetic child's diet.
- Exercise is an essential part of the regimen because it helps to burn up blood sugar instead of storing it as fat, and it in-creases metabolism, thereby preventing obesity.
- Playing sports and working out make your children and you feel better.
- Exercises re-establishes balance in your bodily processes.

We are beset with problems caused by the complexity, stress, and speed of modern life. Our unhealthy responses to these problems and poor health habits are passed on to our kids by the examples we set. Disregard of good health habits results in diseases like Type 2 diabetes, hypertension, heart disease, and cancer. These are not inevitable occurrences, but are directly related to our daily activities, ignorance of preventive measures, and failure to follow—and teach our children to follow—pathways to health. We need to correct the responses that have proved themselves a failure—responses we continue to employ through impatience and lack of imagination and resolve. We need to treat our children with care. The price of carelessness can be very high indeed.

Wendy's Story

Wendy, a 5-year-old, had symptoms of thirst, frequent urination, and nocturnal incontinence, with fatigue and a weight loss of 8 pounds. Her blood sugar was 333, three times normal. After being diagnosed with Type 1 diabetes, she was hospitalized for three days and started on insulin.

The hospital nutritionist told her she could eat anything she wanted. Wendy had only to follow a schedule and consume measured amounts of each carbohydrate, which was assigned a unit value. For lunch, she could eat two carbohydrate units. It didn't matter if those units consisted of white bread, potatoes, apples, ice cream, cake, noodles, or pancakes. Carbohydrate "exchanges" were made to coordinate food intake with insulin dosage in order to control the blood-sugar level. There was no discussion of nutrition or of foods that are beneficial versus those that are not.

Wendy's parents knew that their daughter would be subject to greater health risks than other children, and that those risks would continue in her adult life. They wanted to address all relevant factors and create a program with the most positive impact on her future health. But Wendy's physician and nutritionist had a much more short-term view. They only considered foods from the standpoint of immediate blood-sugar control, ignoring vitamin and mineral content, salt, fiber, and damaging chemical additives in food. They also ignored the possible effects on cholesterol level, blood pressure, and future risk of heart disease and cancer.

Instead of telling Wendy and her parents to measure units of carbohydrates, her nutritionist should have distinguished between simple and complex carbohydrates. Wendy should have been instructed to eat as few simple carbohydrates as possible and as many complex carbohydrates as she wished. The reasons are simple:

- Complex carbohydrates usually require less insulin to control the blood-sugar level than refined carbohydrates. They also contain more fiber and nutrients.
- The less insulin required, the less chance of hypoglycemia.

An hour with my nutritionist helped Wendy's parents to understand the rationale behind our dietary recommendations. As they learned the new system, they saw that Wendy's diabetes could be better controlled with lower doses of insulin and no need to measure food portions. By learning to adapt to staying away from certain foods, Wendy's parents were highly pleased by the results they observed in their daughter: better glucose control and more understanding and peace of mind.

Diet and Blood-Sugar Fluctuations

Parents of diabetic children worry constantly about blood-sugar levels that are too high or too low. A child's blood sugar can go from 40 to 400 and back down to 40 in a single day. These peaks and valleys can be moderated by:

1. Increasing the intake of fiber.
2. Substituting complex for simple and refined carbohydrates.
3. Combining carbohydrates with proteins and good fats in the same meal.

By following these guidelines, you child's blood-sugar levels will stay lower after eating, thus lessening the requirement for insulin.

Exchange Lists—Why You Don't Need Them

Traditional diabetic regimens use exchange lists. This means you are only allowed certain amounts of specific carbohydrates so that your blood sugar won't rise out of control. Values are assigned to ice cream, cookies, soft drinks, bread, and other simple carbohydrates. For instance, if you want to exchange bread for cookies, you need to know how many cookies you can eat without needing to raise the dose of insulin.

Exchange lists require weighing and measuring, and are tedious to use. I don't use them because they are only necessary when you eat high-glycemic-index foods. If you avoid high-glycemic-index foods, your blood-sugar level will not be much affected by what you eat or how much you eat. Foods containing complex carbohydrates or higher quantities of protein and fat (such as nuts and seeds) have a lower glycemic index. Just have an average serving, and your blood sugar will be minimally affected (see page 109 for the glycemic index of common foods).

Making the right food choices spares a lot of mathematical effort. Much damage is done when the nutritional philosophy emphasizes blood-sugar control instead of which foods are eaten. Blood-sugar control is easier with proper dietary choices.

Fiber Helps Control Blood Sugar

Fiber helps control blood sugar by decreasing the rate of carbohydrate absorption from the gastrointestinal tract. Fiber supplements are highly effective and can help diabetics reduce their insulin requirements by about one third. Many people with Type 2 diabetes need not take insulin at all while on a high-fiber diet. The following vegetables, beans, nuts and fruits are particularly high in fiber content:

Vegetable	Grams of Fiber
Black beans, ½ cup	8
Lentils, ½ cup	8
Kidney beans, ½ cup	7
Lima beans, ½ cup	6
Peanuts, ½ cup	6
Chickpeas, ½ cup	5
Potato, baked with skin	5
Oatmeal, 1 cup cooked	4
Wheat germ, ¼ cup	4

Fruit	Grams of Fiber
Apple, with skin	4
Pear, with skin	4
Raspberries, ½ cup	4

NEW STUDY ON FIBER AND TYPE 2 DIABETES

A study reported in *The New England Journal of Medicine* (May 11, 2000; Issue 342, Number 19) reaffirms the value of fiber for treating Type 2 diabetes.

Researchers examined thirteen patients who spent six weeks on a diet that followed the American Dietary Association guidelines and six weeks on a diet that contained significantly more fiber than specified in the guidelines.

When the patients were on the high-fiber diet, their daily plasma glucose concentrations were 10 percent lower, and other measures dropped by similarly significant amounts.

The researchers are from the University of Texas Southwestern Medical Center and the Veterans Affairs Medical Center, both in Dallas.

In an editorial that accompanied their report, Dr. Marc Rendell of the Creighton Diabetes Center in Omaha noted that the improvement was roughly equivalent to the usual effect of adding another drug to the treatment regimen of a diabetic patient.

"It would be more desirable first to take full advantage of the improvements that can be attained by dietary modification," before adding medicine to medicine, Dr. Rendell wrote. (Source: *The New York Times*, May 15, 2000).

The Glycemic Index

Foods are digested and absorbed in the stomach and small intestine. When you eat, your blood sugar rises at a rate mostly dependent on the amount and type of carbohydrates in your food. The glycemic index of a food indicates the degree to which that food raises the blood-sugar level after eating. The higher the glycemic index, the higher the blood sugar goes up.

The following table lists common foods and their glycemic index. Foods with a higher protein and fat content have a lower glycemic index because they tend not to raise the blood sugar. Foods higher in fiber also have a lower glycemic index. Apples, for example, have a lower glycemic index than apple juice, which contains very little fiber.

The lower the glycemic index of the foods you eat, the better. In general, you should try to choose foods that have a glycemic index less than 70.

Using the Glycemic Index

The glycemic index is important because it determines how much insulin will be required to bring the blood sugar back down to normal. With a higher glycemic index, bread and potatoes raise the blood sugar to higher levels and require the release of more insulin.

The result of this increased release of insulin is to make people fatter, raise triglycerides (undesirable since this increases the risk of heart disease), lower HDL (the good cholesterol), and create a situation of insulin resistance leading to diabetes.

A cornerstone of both the prevention and treatment of diabetes mellitus is a diet of low-glycemic-index foods. But it is not necessary to investigate the glycemic index of every food before

GLYCEMIC INDEX—WHITE BREAD STANDARD (WHITE BREAD=100)

Fruits			
Cherries	32	Kiwi	75
Grapefruit	36	Banana	77
Pear	53	Mango	80
Apple	54	Apricot	82
Plum	55	Raisins	91
Peach	60	Pineapple	94
Orange	63	Watermelon	103
Grapes	66	Dates	141

Vegetables			
Green Leafy Vegetables	15	Beets	91
Peas	68	Mashed potato	100
Carrots	70	Pumpkin	107
Yams	73	French fries	107
Sweet potato	77	Instant potato	118
Corn	78	Baked potato	121
New potato	81		

Legumes			
Chana dal (yellow lentils)	12	Lima beans	46
Soybeans	25	Chickpeas	47
Red lentils	36	Navy beans	54
Kidney beans	42	Pinto beans	55
Green lentils	42	Black-eyed beans	59
Butter beans	44		

Breads			
Barley kernel bread	55	Rye flour bread	92
Rye kernel bread	66	Barley flour bread	95
Oat bran bread	68	Whole wheat bread	99
Mixed grain bread	69	White bread	100
Pumpernickel	71	Bagel, white	103
Pita bread	82	Bread stuffing	106
Hamburger bun	87	French baguette	136

Breakfast Cereals			
Rice bran	27	Kellogg's Mini-Wheats	81
Kellogg's All-Bran Fruit 'n Oats	55	Grapenuts	96
Kellogg's Guardian	59	Shredded wheat	99
All-Bran	60	Cream of wheat	100

GLYCEMIC INDEX—WHITE BREAD STANDARD (WHITE BREAD=100)

Red River Cereal	70	Puffed wheat	105
Oatmeal		Cheerios	106
(old-fashioned)	70		
Bran Buds	75	Rice Krispies	117
Special K	77	Corn Chex	118
Oat Bran	78	Corn Flakes	119
Kellogg's Honey		Crispix	124
Smacks	78		
Muesli	80	RiceChex	127

Cereal Grains

Barley, pearled	36	Rice, white	83
Rye	48	Couscous	93
Wheat kernels	59	Barley, rolled	94
Bulgur	68	Cornmeal	98
Barley, cracked	72	Millet	101
Buckwheat	78	Rice, instant	128
Rice, brown	79		

Soups

Tomato soup	54	Split pea soup	86
Lentil soup	63	Black bean soup	92

Sugars

Fructose	32	Sucrose	92
Lactose	65	Glucose	137
Honey	83	Maltose	150
High-fructose syrup	89		

Pasta

Fettucine	46	Linguini	65
Vermicelli	50	Gnocchi	95
Spaghetti	59	Rice pasta, brown	131
Macaroni	64		

Bakery Products

Cake, sponge	66	Croissants	96
Pastry	84	Doughnut	108
Pizza, cheese	86	Waffles	109
Muffins	88		

you offer it to your child. If you look through the charts, you will see that certain groups of foods are more acceptable than others. Refined carbohydrates always have a higher glycemic index than the natural foods they come from. For example, whole grains are preferable to bread and cold cereals made from these grains because the refining process ensures that they will provoke elevated blood sugars. Similarly, juices will always have a higher glycemic index than the fruits from which they come because fiber is lost in the extraction process. Regarding fruits, tropical fruits such as pineapple, banana, mango, papaya, and kiwi have a high glycemic index and should be avoided. Cherries and berries, on the other hand, have a low glycemic index and can be eaten. Foods either made from sugar—candy, soft drinks—or foods with sugar added—baked goods, cereals—will have a high glycemic index. Foods high in protein or fat—nuts, seeds, beans and lentils—tend to have a lower glycemic index. Best of all are green vegetables.

If high-glycemic-index foods are desired, they can be consumed with low-glycemic-index foods so that the collective effect on blood-sugar elevation is reduced. For instance, mashed potatoes (high glycemic index) can be eaten with chicken and broccoli (low glycemic index).

The Glycemic Index Is Not the Ten Commandments

The glycemic index is an advisory for proper food choices, not the sole standard of meal planning. Remember that foods with a higher glycemic index may prove to be healthier for diabetics and overweight people than foods with a lower glycemic index. For example, carrots have a higher glycemic index than spaghetti. Spaghetti, however, is much denser in calories. To get 50 grams of sugar from carrots, you would have to consume more than a pound of this vegetable, which would come to only 220 calories. A pound of spaghetti provides 600 calories and 130 grams of sugar. Thus, there's a much greater chance of gaining weight from eating spaghetti than carrots. In addition, some high-glycemic-index foods are healthier because they contain more nutrients, less fat, and no harmful additives or preservatives.

Other factors than the glycemic index come into play when making food choices. Water, for example, is always the preferred beverage when you are trying to lose weight, no matter what the glycemic index of the drink you choose. Whole milk has a low glycemic index (less than 40), but a quart of milk still contains 630 calories. Water, on the other hand, has no calories. By drinking a quart of water instead of milk every day, you would lose more than a pound a week.

Using the glycemic index allows you to offset one high-index food with several low-index foods, and I highly recommend such "creative accounting." Combining carrots with peas and broccoli, for example, results in a lower glycemic index than carrots alone. Combining calorie-rich foods with low-calorie foods results in fewer weight problems. For instance, if you add mushrooms, asparagus, zucchini, and herbs to spaghetti, you have a much safer food than spaghetti with cream sauce. In addition, the glycemic index can save you from the effects of unknowingly eating several high-index foods together.

Although the list of foods in the glycemic index may look a bit daunting at first, you will quickly catch on to the thinking behind it and be able to make your own judgments concerning the values of foods not included. Accuracy of assigning percentage points is much less important than gaining an overall understanding of foods and insulin response.

Making the Index Work for You

- Even when processed carbohydrates belong in the same glycemic-index category as whole-grain products, they are less beneficial because they lack the vitamins, minerals, and fiber that whole-grain foods possess.
- When proteins and fats (meat, chicken, fish, beans, nuts) are eaten with high- or moderate-glycemic foods, they help slow down absorption of carbohydrates, therefore helping to prevent sharp rises in blood-sugar and insulin levels.
- Remember that the kind of energy you feel is closely tied to

this index. The higher the food on the glycemic index, the faster the burst of energy and the sooner the letdown.

- Foods that have a lower glycemic index value increasingly provide a healthier, more long-term kind of energy.
- Refined or processed foods always have a higher glycemic index than the natural foods they came from.
- Fruit juices have a higher glycemic index than the whole fruits they come from.
- White bread has a very high glycemic index, and whole-grain bread isn't much better.
- Breakfast cereals are made from highly processed grains and have a glycemic index even higher than bread.
- Instant cooked cereal and instant rice have high-glycemic-index numbers.
- Since fiber is lost with heating, the longer a food is cooked, the higher its glycemic number. For example, noodles al dente do not raise blood sugar as much as noodles cooked till they are soft.
- Baked potatoes have a high-glycemic-index number. You can lessen this by combining them with foods having a low-glycemic-index number such as beans or lentils.
- The fact that an esteemed, wealthy, and talented athlete or movie star endorses a product does not make it more acceptable for a diabetic or an overweight child.

Our knowledge of the effect of high-glycemic-index foods on insulin production and body weight enables us to see how changes in the American diet over the last 20 years have led to an alarming increase in serious obesity problems, including heart disease and Type 2 diabetes. To reduce heart disease, many of us have made a massive effort to eliminate fat from our diet. Food companies responded by concocting refined foods that were lower in fat but were loaded with sugar. Now the average American consumes 150 pounds of sugar a year, almost half a pound a day. Cholesterol levels have come down, but we have instead a resounding escalation of obesity and Type 2 diabetes.

Overcoming Dietary Misinformation

I have often seen diabetic children who were eating cold cereals and drinking fruit juice. When I asked their parents about this, they said they were told these foods were acceptable. That is far from the truth. This misinformation comes from caregivers who don't thoroughly understand the role of nutrition, supplements, and exercise in treating and preventing diabetes. While some health-care professionals are uninformed, others believe that most parents of diabetic children aren't capable of understanding or adhering to what's involved in controlling the condition. Look what happened to one family when they were given incorrect advice.

Peter's Story

Peter was nine years old when he came from Hawaii to see me in February 1998. Diabetes had been diagnosed one month earlier, when he developed symptoms of weakness, excessive urination, and weight loss. The day he entered the hospital, Peter was suffering from severe abdominal pain, vomiting, lethargy and dehydration. He had lost eight pounds. His blood sugar was very high, over 700, and he had early ketoacidosis. He stayed in the hospital five days, initially in the intensive care unit, receiving intravenous fluids and insulin. He was discharged on two doses of insulin a day. The dose was gradually reduced because of repeated hypoglycemic reactions.

Standing at Peter's bedside in the intensive care unit, his physician offered Peter's mother a litany of diabetic complications, including amputation. This frightened Peter's mother even more. When asked about diet, the doctor said Peter could eat anything he wanted, as long as he took his insulin. Peter's mother knew this wasn't right. She then asked about giving her son nutritional supplements and was told she could give him whatever she liked.

Later she took Peter to another diabetes specialist, looking for answers. She asked him about the benefits of nutritional supplements for diabetics. He became irate. He told her that she was a selfish and terrible mother who was only thinking of herself.

He said her behavior was a form of child abuse. He was against the use of supplements. Subsequently he wrote an article about her in a local newspaper, describing parents who look for "miracle cures" for their children. Yet she was not looking for a miracle cure, only for whatever information she could find to help her son manage his illness.

When Peter arrived at my office, he was already taking nutritional supplements in large amounts. His blood had fallen to the point where he no longer required insulin. He had entered the honeymoon phase, the time early in the course of Type 1 diabetes when insulin production has risen high enough to permit satisfactory blood-sugar control with little or no additional insulin. The supplements likely supported this improvement.

Our nutritionist provided dietary information. Peter's previous diet had included cold cereals, brown sugar, honey, orange juice, chocolate, doughnuts, frozen yogurt, and ice cream. These high-glycemic-index foods were replaced with safer, low-glycemic-index alternatives.

The supplements I recommended were multivitamins, niacinamide, biotin, chromium, vanadium, coenzyme Q-10, lipoic acid, N-acetyl cysteine, and grapeseed extract.

Peter's mother contacted me several times after they returned home. Peter's insulin requirement remained minimal for many months, usually 3–4 units a day. He was very sensitive to insulin, with episodes of hypoglycemia when only one extra unit of insulin was given. His glucose level would rise if he ate candy or got upset.

I last spoke to Peter's mother in December 1999, when he was 11 years old. He has seen a physician only once since his visit here. It was hard finding a physician that he and his mother liked. Peter regularly tested his blood sugars, before each meal and at bedtime. He drew up and administered his insulin before each meal. Sometimes he had trouble injecting the insulin and felt frustrated. One day he protested to his mother, "You don't know what it's like." He apologized to her a few hours later.

Peter was eating papaya (a tropical fruit with a high glycemic index that we do not recommend) for breakfast. His 14-year-old brother Kip had become very diet-conscious, since he had a rising interest in sports and girls. Kip was setting a good example for Peter. Peter often did not eat the lunch his mother prepared for him on schooldays, so she started giving him some higher glycemic-index foods, or a Balance Bar. She knew this wasn't the best diet, but Peter was playing a lot of sports, and she was afraid of hypoglycemia if he missed eating lunch.

Peter now injected a total of twelve units of insulin daily, still a low dose. Despite some family problems (his parents were separated), he was usually in good spirits. With the instruction and support of his mother, Peter understood his illness and was able to follow most of the rules and to avoid serious problems. I was not worried about his future. His mother's love was unconditional, and that is a valuable asset to have when confronting diabetes.

Every child and every family has a different experience with diabetes. It is never easy, but it is much easier when basic nutritional principles are understood and accepted, when the child actively participates and has some responsibility for his own care, when the family is supportive and sets a good example. Changes at home and in school offer challenges that require new adjustments.

It is imperative that every physician involved in a child's care be understanding and sympathetic. A physician who depicts a negative prognosis to parents who are already terrified is doing them a disservice. The physician's objective should not be to create fear and trembling in order to bring about compliance. The offer of good health and freedom from complications is a better motivator. Education and self-sufficiency offer the greatest empowerment.

There are times when living with diabetes is a great imposition. The onset of puberty, with its physical and emotional changes, is an especially trying period. But the same rules apply: The child should retain responsibility for his own care. Parent and child should maintain strong communication. Family support should be constant.

Parents are usually willing to eliminate sugars and simple carbohydrates from their children's diet when they learn that the results will be a steadier blood-sugar level and fewer episodes of the irritability and fatigue typical of hypoglycemic reactions. I find that such parents readily understand what's involved. Once they do, they are dedicated, intelligent advocates fighting for their children's lives. Fortunately for Peter and other children like him, the parents had doubts about the information they were given and brought their children to our clinic to try a new approach.

Managing Diabetes Takes Work

Having treated children with diabetes and worked with worried, dedicated parents to get their children healthy, I know firsthand that it's far from easy to manage diabetes or to prevent or reverse obesity. Nor is it cheap. It's time-consuming, requiring constant vigilance and strong motivation. It is, in short, like any other form of education.

But gradually the effort and training pay off as parent and child apply what they have learned. Tastes can be refined and desires modified. Children can learn to choose the right foods, help shop for them, and prepare them. They can learn that certain foods make them sick. And they can help their parents follow the rules, too. Even in families where everyone is already fat, change is possible.

Major problems exist, however, in societies beset by false information, because that information has to be discarded before truthful information can be applied. In the United States, the food industry earns a trillion dollars a year. It's a business that sells all kinds of foods, good and bad, often indiscriminately. Supermarkets don't have signs reading *Good Foods Here* and *Bad Foods Here*. In fact, it often seems that the foods that are least healthy receive the most marketing. The soft-drink industry, offering no good nutrition, spends billions of dollars a year promoting its products. Over the years, advertising pays off. Cold cereal for breakfast becomes a tradition. So does coffee and a sweet roll in the morning, beer during ball games, and popcorn doused with butter during movies.

Fast-food businesses also spend billions on advertising, especially on children's television shows and on huge billboards and large, flashy signs sporting logos readily identifiable to millions of kids. Fast foods taste good. They are full of salt, sugar, and fat—and children get accustomed to that taste. Children also like the prizes they receive and the bonus goodies.

Because fast foods are fast, they've become part of the American lifestyle, a quick fix for parents who have too many roles to juggle. Convenience is very important here. There's no shopping, no preparation, and no cleaning up afterward. You go in, you order, and you eat—and it's fairly cheap. Dozens of people in the restaurants look just like you and your kids, so it is socially acceptable. What you hear, read, and see all indicate that this activity is the norm.

Because there's no law requiring health warnings for foods, what you do not hear, read, or see is that people who are overweight or diabetic or who have heart disease or hypertension may be damaged by this product. Fast food has become almost synonymous with life in the twenty-first century, a feat accomplished at enormous expense by businessmen whose purpose has been not to create a healthy society, but to make money.

Advertising slogans repeated often enough acquire a patina of truth. I believe that such endless promotions are nefarious. Some people might say that this is the necessary price we must pay for free speech. However, if we must allow the proliferation of false information, we should also make the truth available by teaching good nutrition in our schools. Our government should subsidize nutritional education and provide healthy and tasty meals in public institutions. In the end, the cost for these programs would probably be less than we pay for the diseases we are creating through misinformation and ignorance.

CHAPTER 7

Exercise and Supplements

Exercise May Be More Important Than Diet

There are compelling reasons to get your diabetic child and the rest of your family involved in exercise. Physical activity is the single most important factor in eliminating Type 2 diabetes and decreasing the need for supplemental insulin in Type 1 diabetes. It is also key in preventing Type 2 diabetes because it helps to eliminate obesity, a major factor in the development of the disease.

Physical activity is a major factor influencing the accumulation and distribution of body fat, especially in those with a genetic predisposition to be fat. A study published in the *Annals of Internal Medicine* in 1999 detailed the effect of physical activity on body fat in female twins genetically predisposed to having similar physical characteristics. The twins who participated in vigorous weight-bearing activities had less abdominal fat and, depending on their level of exercise, weighed 9 to 12 pounds less than their overweight, sedentary twins. Differences became more dramatic as the amount of exercise increased. The study showed dramatically that exercise is a deterrent to obesity even in obese families.

Even more startling is the study's finding that exercise is the single most effective factor in preventing obesity—significantly more important than reducing caloric intake or total dietary fat. In fact, the researchers found that reductions in neither caloric intake nor dietary fat had any effect on total body fat compared to increases in physical activity.

Look at the effect that getting involved with exercise had on 17-year-old Kara, whose story was told at the beginning of this book.

Kara Revisited

After she fell out of a tree at age 13 and broke her leg, Kara had to give up tap dancing and ballet, which had kept her fit and healthy. She became almost totally inactive and gained an enormous amount of weight as the result of her fast-food diet and her lack of exercise.

By the time Kara was 17, she weighed 170 pounds. She was diagnosed as having Syndrome X, a combination of Type 2 diabetes, high cholesterol, and high triglycerides. Unless she made some major lifestyle changes, her future would likely include high blood pressure, gout, and cardiovascular disease.

I saw Kara when she was 17. After she understood the need for regular physical activity to control her weight and increase the effectiveness of her body's insulin, Kara joined a bicycle club. She also started taking the nutritional supplements we prescribed, including multivitamins and minerals, with special formulations of essential fatty acids, chromium, vanadium, alpha lipoic acid, and gymnema sylvestre (I will discuss these later on).

Within a few months, Kara became as fanatic about cycling as she had once been about dancing. As a result of cycling 200 miles a week, she lost 40 pounds; her blood sugar fell to normal, as did her triglycerides and cholesterol.

Given the genetic tendency for diabetes she'd inherited, I explained that if Kara stopped exercising, started eating the wrong foods again, and gained weight, the disease could just as easily reassert itself.

Since Type 2 diabetes is closely correlated with obesity, you might expect that lack of exercise would increase the likelihood of developing diabetes, as it did in Kara's case. That is, in fact, just how the obesity-diabetes connection works. According to a 1999 study by Ming Wei and co-workers in the *Annals of Internal Medicine* ("The Association Between Cardiorespiratory Fitness and Impaired Fasting Glucose and Type II Diabetes Mellitus in Men," 1999; 130: 89–96), men who were not physically fit had twice the incidence of mild blood-sugar elevations, and almost four times the incidence of confirmed diabetes as men at the highest level of fitness.

In the same study, researchers found that a lack of physical activity contributes to mortality in individuals with Type 2 diabetes. Over a 12-year period, physically inactive men had almost twice the risk of dying compared with men who engaged in active exercise programs. In addition, men who were physically unfit (determined by their limited ability to perform on a treadmill) had over twice the mortality risk of men with a higher exercise capacity. These findings held even after adjustment for obesity, high glucose levels, and high blood pressure. Thus, diabetics who establish active exercise programs can double their chances of survival.

Regular exercise:

- Prevents diabetes by enhancing insulin activity.
- Increases blood flow and insulin supply to muscle tissues.
- Promotes the entry of glucose into muscle cells through a mechanism separate from the action of insulin.
- Improves blood-sugar control in those who already have diabetes by reducing the amount of insulin or other drugs needed to restore normal blood-sugar levels.
- Raises the level of HDL (good cholesterol) and thus lowers the risk of heart disease. The more hours you run, the higher your HDL goes.
- Reduces blood pressure, another risk factor for heart disease and stroke. A study of Japanese men in Osaka showed that the more time they spent walking to work, the less chance they had of developing high blood pressure. Apparently, in Japan, walking to work is the only exercise many men get. Even mild exercise lowers blood pressure, and does so in people who have either normal or elevated blood pressure.

If these reasons aren't persuasive enough, consider the fact that people who are sedentary have a 30 to 125 percent higher risk of diabetes than those who are physically active.

EXERCISE LOWERS LEVEL OF FAT HORMONE

A study conducted at the Harvard School of Public Health has found that physically active people have lower blood levels of the hormone leptin. First identified in 1994, leptin has been dubbed the "fat" hormone because it is produced by the body's fat cells. It is highest in people who are overweight, don't exercise, and eat foods that are high in saturated fats and cholesterol.

Leptin may be involved in the relation between diabetes and obesity by playing a role in the insulin resistance caused by obesity. A team of scientists at the University of Texas Southwestern Medical Center have reported that leptin, found in greater quantity in obese subjects, caused insulin-producing pancreatic cells to die, resulting in Type 2 diabetes. Not only do overweight men have higher leptin levels than thin men, but so do men with insulin resistance and a tendency to become diabetic.

The good news, as shown by the Harvard study, is that exercise is an effective way to dramatically lower leptin levels in the blood.

Get Your Family Moving!

Exercise is not just good for the body. It also helps to build up neurological connections in a child's brain. Vision, hearing, tactility, coordination, and intelligence are improved by all forms of physical activity. To reap the benefits of exercise:

- Encourage your kids to play sports daily.
- Set a good example for your children by participating in physical activities regularly.
- Make sports and working-out a part of your family's life. Playing sports with your kids will strengthen your relationship with them and very likely provide you with some of the greatest pleasures of your life.
- Start kids playing sports early, setting up a pattern of physi-

cal activity for a lifetime. People who never got involved in sports in their youth often find them boring and difficult when they get older.

- Encourage an interest in non-contact sports like gymnastics, swimming, running, climbing, handball, golf, tennis, rollerblading, bicycling, ice skating, and canoeing. This will ensure that kids who don't like the rough and tumble of physical contact can still exercise (just be sure they wear the appropriate protective clothing).
- Don't forget dancing. It's fun and it surpasses many sports in promoting cardiovascular fitness and weight control.
- Consider yoga and tai-chi, which offer profound benefits for physical conditioning and stress reduction.

Exercise and Insulin

When exercising, diabetic children require special attention. First of all, changes should be made in how insulin is given. Instead of administering the required doses of insulin into the thigh, injections should be given in the abdominal area. That's because insulin given by injection into the thigh is absorbed into the bloodstream more quickly than usual because of increased blood flow to thigh tissues during exercise.

Exercise lowers the blood sugar by increasing blood flow to the muscles and promoting the entry of glucose into the cells. Thus, it decreases insulin requirements. Unless insulin dosages are properly reduced, diabetics can experience hypoglycemic reactions. Glucose tablets should always be available in case hypoglycemia occurs. These tablets raise a low blood-sugar level within minutes.

How do you go about reducing the need for insulin safely? Because few of us can predict the effect of a particular activity on the blood-sugar level, when a diabetic child begins exercising or changes sports, it's smart to take frequent readings of blood sugar and record the response to exercise in a diary. For example, the insulin dose prior to a game of soccer may need to be decreased 50 percent or more. Such prolonged, vigorous physical activity greatly promotes the uptake of glucose by skeletal muscle. When I was a child, the third baseman on my favorite baseball team took insulin for his diabetes and had to cut his dose almost completely before ball games. Diabetic athletes often need to lower their insulin on days when they compete in order to avoid hypoglycemic reactions.

Before exercise, it is often desirable to reduce the dose of insulin because lower doses reduce the risk of hypoglycemic reactions and permit smoother control of blood sugar. That's why exercise is so vital. As body fat is reduced and muscle bulk increased with exercise, resistance to the action of insulin and the required dose of insulin will both diminish. When a diabetic has a daily exercise program in place, she may be able to eliminate a scheduled dose of insulin, thus simplifying the management of the disease. In my experience, the combination of regular exercise, improved diet, weight loss, and nutritional supplementation reduces insulin requirements by at least 30 percent in Type 1 diabetics. For Type 2 diabetics who are treated with either insulin or oral hypoglycemic agents, those medications can sometimes be completely eliminated.

TENNIS AWARDS

The Donnelly Awards of $5,000 are awarded annually to two tennis players age 14 to 21 who have Type 1 diabetes. The Billie Jean King Foundation, in cooperation with the American Diabetes Association, presents the awards at a late-summer World Team Tennis event.

The awards are in honor of two sisters who were diagnosed with Type 1 diabetes as young children. Despite their illness, they went on to compete in tennis at the national level. They earned full athletic scholarships at Northwestern and the University of Iowa.

For information about the awards, contact World Team Tennis at (312) 245-5300 or *www.worldteam tennis.com*.

Get in the Exercise Habit Early

It's never too early to get children involved in exercise and sports, as a four-year study by the National Heart, Lung and Blood Institute illustrates. From 1991 to 1994, third graders at fifty-six elementary schools in four states took part in a food and fitness behaviors study organized by the Institute. They ate school lunches lower in fat, participated in moderate to vigorous exercise classes, and took part in health classes, some of which involved their parents.

In a follow-up study published in 1999, researchers evaluated 73 percent of the children in the original program after they had moved on to middle schools that did not provide the program. The children were still eating a healthier diet and leading a more active life than children who had been in the original control groups.

This pleased the lead researcher, Dr. Philip R. Nader, professor of pediatrics at the University of California at San Diego, who published the study in the July 1999 issue of *Archives of Pediatric and Adolescent Medicine*. "The thing that encouraged us is that kids are still reporting that they have healthy diets and do more activity," he said.

The moral? Gloria Olivas Levins, principal of an El Paso elementary school in the program, puts it best: "The children have become much more aware of their eating habits and exercise." She added, "The program has an impact on our staff. Even me."

SPORTS MAKE YOUR FAMILY HEALTHIER

If you make exercise part of your daily life, your family will experience many rewards:

- Overweight children will slim down.
- Type 2 diabetes will be prevented.
- Type 1 diabetes will become better controlled and insulin doses lowered.
- Risks of developing hypertension and heart disease will be minimized.
- The whole family will feel better.
- Attitude and self-image will improve.

The Role of Supplements

Supplements are an essential component of my program. Though recommendations vary with diagnosis, severity of illness, and age, in general, I recommend a regular program of comprehensive vitamin and mineral supplementation. The time is long gone when supplements were intended only to prevent diseases due to deficiency states. We know now that vitamin C in an amount beyond that which prevents scurvy works to reduce blood pressure, support immune system function, and prevent cardiac disease. Supplemental folic acid lowers the incidence of serious neurologic birth defects. Zinc speeds recovery from respiratory infections, as does vitamin A. Standard medical textbooks now emphasize the use of supplements not simply to prevent deficiency states, but to establish optimal physiologic function. Unfortunately, many traditional physicians have yet to accept this new paradigm.

The following is a list, prepared by the Food and Nutrition Board, of Recommended Daily Allowances (RDAs) for nutrients suggested for children. Do not assume they are provided in your child's diet, even if it is a good diet. You cannot know the nutrient concentrations in the soil used to grow these foods. If your child has a diet full of refined foods and fast foods, you can be assured that nutrient deficiencies exist. Remember that vitamins and minerals are not drugs. They rarely have side effects.

Other trace minerals are necessary, but the minimum daily requirement has not been ascertained. These include manganese (probably 10 mg), chromium (probably 200 mcg), selenium (probably 200 mcg), and molybdenum (about 125 mcg).

The requirements for essential fatty acids are about 3 grams for omega-3 fatty acids and 3 grams for omega-6 fatty acids.

Larger amounts of certain nutrients are advised for diabetics (both Type 1 and Type 2), including vitamin C, vitamin E, magnesium, trace minerals, and others. Diabetics derive additional benefits from antioxidants and essential fatty acids that help prevent tissue deterioration, and minerals that enhance the action of insulin. Specific doses of these nutrients are discussed in this chapter.

	1 to 4 Years Old	Over 4 to Adult
Vitamin A	2500 units	5000 units
Vitamin C	40 mg	60 mg
Thiamin (B_1)	1 mg	2 mg
Riboflavin (B_2)	1 mg	2 mg
Niacin	10 mg	20 mg
Pantothenic acid	5 mg	10 mg
Vitamin B_6	1 mg	2 mg
Vitamin B_{12}	3 mcg	6 mcg
Folic acid	200 mcg	400 mcg
Biotin	150 mcg	300 mcg
Vitamin D	400 units	400 units
Vitamin E	10 units	30 units
Vitamin K	80 mcg	80 mcg
Zinc	8 mg	15 mg
Copper	1 mg	2 mg
Magnesium	200 mg	400 mg
Iodine	75 mcg	75 mcg
Calcium	800 mg	800 mg, males
		1200 mg, females

1 mg = 1 milligram, one thousandth of a gram. There are thirty grams in one ounce.

1 mcg = 1 microgram, one millionth of a gram, or one thousandth of a milligram.

Special Nutrients for Diabetic Children

Certain nutrients offer particular benefits to diabetics. These nutrients include essential fatty acids, B vitamins, antioxidant vitamins C and E, magnesium, coenzyme Q10, lipoic acid, chromium, and vanadium. Adding them to a diabetic's diet, along with exercise, stress reduction, and dietary changes, can make a radical difference in a diabetic's health. These nutrients can improve blood-sugar control and lower insulin requirements, as well as lower the risk of future complications. They can also improve one's sense of well-being. Case in point: 16-year-old Grant.

Grant's Story

Diagnosed with Type 1 diabetes, Grant had the classic diabetic symptoms of excessive thirst and urination plus a nine-pound weight loss. His blood sugar was 220, twice the normal amount. His doctors started him on the short-acting insulin Humalog with each meal and the long-acting insulin Ultralente twice a day for a total of 36 units daily. His diet was changed to low-glycemic foods (see chapter 6), which excluded cold cereals, bread, soft drinks, and other items that elevate blood sugar levels quickly and require higher doses of insulin.

When he came to our clinic, Grant was started on nutritional supplements, including chromium, magnesium, and lipoic acid. He also took Muraglycine, a highly concentrated extract obtained from a bacterium called lactobacillus bulgaricus. Muraglycine is a strong potentiator of insulin activity. It is now available as a food supplement called Leukomeal (further information can be found on my website, *www.allansosinmd.com*).

As a result of this program, Grant's insulin dose was gradually reduced to 25 units a day. However, his blood-sugar level still fell too low, and his insulin dose was reduced even more. We further modified his diet to increase protein and limit simple carbohydrates. His insulin dose had to be cut again. His nutritional supplements included the following:

Lipoic acid, 150 mg
Coenzyme Q10, 100 mg
Magnesium, 1,000 mg
Vanadyl sulfate, 50 mg
Gymnema sylvestre, 200 mg
Chromium picolinate, 600 mcg
Biotin, 8 mg
Flaxseed oil, 1 tablespoon
Leukomeal (Muraglycine), 10 mg

Because several herbs are effective in enhancing insulin activity and are safe to use, we also started him on leaf extract from the herb Gymnema sylvestre, which enhances insulin action. Gymnema sylvestre is so effective that we prescribe it most often.

Six weeks after Grant began taking these supplements, his blood sugar had come down to normal levels. He was able to completely stop using insulin. Although this improvement was temporary, and Grant had to resume insulin therapy, the dose he needed was significantly lower than he had taken previously.

Making the "honeymoon" last longer

Grant's experience was typical of the "honeymoon period," a stage that frequently occurs after the onset of Type 1 diabetes, when the pancreas sometimes recovers its ability to produce insulin. Although the need for insulin often resurfaces several months later, it's possible to prolong this honeymoon period and reduce future insulin requirements by empowering the action of insulin. This can be done through supplements, a low-glycemic diet, and regular exercise.

Antioxidants

Our bodies use oxygen to produce energy. The energy-producing process results in the formation of molecular fragments called oxygen free radicals. Free radicals can react with body tissues and drastically alter their structure and function, usually for the worse. Many experts think that the harmful new compounds formed by free radicals cause physical aging. Free radicals also seem to be associated with cancer and heart disease, and to have a role in diseases typical of aging, such as Alzheimer's, Parkinson's, cataracts, arthritis, and Type 2 diabetes.

Antioxidants join chemically with free radicals in the body, neutralizing their activity. They thus deprive free radicals of the chance to form harmful compounds. We get antioxidants chiefly from fresh fruit and vegetables. When your diet is deficient in fresh fruit and vegetables, you need antioxidant supplements. Vitamins C and E, coenzyme Q10, and lipoic acid are particularly valuable antioxidants for young people with diabetes. Higher doses of antioxidants, taken as supplements, offer further protection against free-radical damage. It is not practical to obtain these higher doses just by eating foods.

Vitamin C

The RDA (recommended daily allowance) of several nutrients, especially vitamin C, is thought to be too low. Recent research indicates that 200 milligrams of vitamin C per day should be the minimum intake. Under certain circumstances, such as infection and after surgery, higher doses are in order. Children under 6 with infections should receive 100 mg per hour while awake. For children over 6, the dose should be 200 mg per hour. Vitamin C also serves as an antioxidant, thus preventing tissue damage. The vitamin C concentration in the brain is 15 times higher than in the rest of the body, and serves to prevent oxidative injury to sensitive neurons. Since diabetics are subject to accelerated oxidative damage, supplemental vitamin C should be provided. Diabetic children under 6 should routinely receive 200 mg per day. Those over 6 should receive 500 mg per day, and those over 12 should receive 1000 mg per day.

Vitamin E

Vitamin E includes the tocopherols and tocotrienols, which are very potent antioxidants. By preventing the oxidation of unsaturated fats, vitamin E protects the lipid (fat) membranes of cells from damage. Nerve cells, red and white blood cells, and lung cells have a high unsaturated fatty acid content and high exposure to oxygen. They are thus very susceptible to oxidation and benefit from increased levels of vitamin E. Vitamin E also prevents vitamin A oxidation and is itself regenerated by vitamin C. Each of the antioxidant vitamins sustains the activity of the others. This is why they should be supplemented together. When you take one antioxidant without the others, you're not getting the full benefit.

D-alpha tocopherol is the most potent natural form of vitamin E, although beta, gamma, and delta tocopherols are also active. Synthetic vitamin E, called dl-alpha tocopherol, is less desirable because it contains the ineffective l-form.

Vitamin E supplementation is valuable in combating excessive oxidation of fatty acids, which is a major cause of tissue damage in diabetics. Excessive oxidation of fatty acids affects:

- Eyes: cataract formation and retinopathy
- Nerves: tingling, numbness, and pain
- Muscles: weakness and atrophy
- Immune system: increased susceptibility to infection

Vitamin E also helps with other disorders in which excessive oxidation of fatty acids is typical, such as multiple sclerosis, Parkinson's disease, Alzheimer's disease, and peripheral neuropathy.

Vitamin E is present in fruits, grains, seeds (especially sunflower seeds), nuts (particularly almonds), and wheat-germ oil, its most concentrated form. But when these foods are processed, vitamin E is lost and the natural unsaturated fats are damaged.

Because the cooking process destroys vitamin E, animal products are poor sources of the vitamin. Food processing, such as the milling of grains to make bread, also destroys vitamin E.

Diabetic children should take supplements of d-alpha tocopherol or mixed tocopherols daily with meals to enhance absorption. I recommend the following dosages:

- Under age 6, 100 iu per day
- 6 to 12, 400 iu per day
- 13 and over, 800 iu per day
- Doses should be increased for children who have neurologic or eye problems to 800–1,200 iu per day
- Adults with these conditions should up their intake to 2,000 iu per day

Coenzyme Q10

CoQ10 lowers blood sugar in diabetics and can also help prevent or treat the many cardiovascular complications that diabetics experience. It is also an intrinsic component of aerobic (requiring oxygen) metabolism in mitochondria, the tiny energy factories within cells. Tissues with more concentrated mitochondria, such as heart muscle, contain much higher levels of CoQ10. Studies have shown that CoQ10 is highly effective in treating cardiac disorders, including congestive heart failure, cardiomyopathy (weakness of the heart muscle), irregular rhythms, and atherosclerosis. It lowers blood pressure, supports immune-system function, and is used as a nutritional aid to people with cancer or chronic fatigue syndrome. It has dramatically improved gum disease.

An antioxidant, CoQ10 helps regenerate vitamin E from its oxidized form and thus participates in the body's complex system of interlacing antioxidants. In this chemical cooperative, each antioxidant helps regenerate the other antioxidants. Thus, the body's supply of these crucial materials is maintained, and they can continue to protect tissues from damage without having to be constantly repleted.

I recommend the following dosages for diabetic children:

• Under age 6, 30 mg per day
• Over 6, 60 mg per day
• Teenagers, 100 mg per day.
• Those with diabetic complications, at least 200–300 mg per day

CoQ10 is not toxic. Because it's absorbed better with a fatty meal or some flaxseed oil, I suggest giving it to children with breakfast, along with their essential fatty acid supplement.

Lipoic acid

Five years ago, hardly any of us had heard of alpha lipoic acid. It was mentioned obscurely as something possibly beneficial for liver failure caused by mushroom poisoning. Today, we know that, like CoQ10, alpha lipoic acid (for simplification, I'll call it simply lipoic acid from here on) is an intrinsic part of energy-producing cellular activities. Like CoQ10 and vitamins A, C, and E, lipoic acid is an antioxidant and helps regenerate other antioxidants. Lipoic acid protects our body cells, but our body manufactures it in very small amounts.

This nutrient is especially critical for diabetics because it increases the uptake and utilization of glucose, and improves blood-sugar control in both Type 1 and Type 2 diabetes. Glycation, the process by which glucose combines with proteins, is a major cause of tissue destruction in diabetics, resulting in neuropathy, kidney damage, and retinal injury that can lead to blindness. Lipoic acid blocks these conditions, while protecting and healing injuries to the eyes, kidneys, and nerves. Diabetics are deficient in lipoic acid, and it is very important for them to receive it as a supplement. As with all the other supplements discussed here, there are no significant side effects associated with its use.

In its antioxidant role, lipoic acid reduces fatty acid oxidation, alterations in the structure of lipids (fats) that result in degeneration and impaired function. When these changes affect cholesterol and other fats called lipoproteins, blood vessels are damaged and atherosclerosis occurs. Thus, lipoic acid may be useful in the prevention and treatment of heart disease.

To ensure adequate levels of lipoic acid, I recommend the following doses for diabetic children:

- Under age 6, 50 mg per day
- 6 to 12, 100 mg per day
- 13 and over, 150 mg per day

If the blood sugar level remains high after one month, raise the dose of lipoic acid an additional 100 mg for each age group.

For individuals with neuropathy or retinopathy, a dose of 600–900 mg per day is recommended.

Magnesium

Magnesium is an essential mineral for more than 100 enzyme systems and a multitude of other physiologic functions. It is plentiful in green vegetables, whole grains, nuts, legumes, and seafood. Most people do not ingest the recommended minimal intake of 400 mg a day. Magnesium is found mainly within cells. Therefore depletion may exist even when serum levels are normal. Magnesium controls blood pressure, regulates cardiac rhythm, prevents muscle cramps and seizures, diminishes allergic symptoms and asthma, and relieves insomnia and anxiety. It participates in the metabolism of glucose and is required for the synthesis of fatty acids and proteins. Symptoms of vomiting, diarrhea, sweating, and excessive urination, such as in uncontrolled diabetes, deplete the body's store of magnesium. Low serum magnesium has been found to be a strong and independent predictor for development of Type 2 diabetes. Individuals with the lowest magnesium levels have twice the risk of developing diabetes as those with the highest levels. Magnesium facilitates the action of insulin and acts as an enzyme co-factor in carbohydrate metabolism. Deficiency may interfere with the binding of insulin to its receptor on cell membranes, suppress the insulin-signaling pathway, or slow glucose metabolism. ("Serum and Dietary Magnesium and the Risk for Type II Diabetes Mellitus," *Archives of Internal Medicine,* vol. 159, Oct. 1, 1999, pp. 2151–2159).

High blood sugar results in excessive urinary losses of magnesium. Magnesium depletion causes elevated blood pressure, vascular spasm, irregular heart rhythm, and neurological dysfunction, increasing the cardiac and neurologic problems to which diabetics are so susceptible.

I have seen cardiac arrhythmias and high blood pressure resolve quickly with magnesium. One of the major benefits of chelation therapy (an intravenous infusion used to treat cardiovascular disorders) is the repletion of magnesium stores. Patients with poor circulation to their legs have noted improved color and warmth in their feet within hours of treatment.

Too much magnesium can cause diarrhea, but it is otherwise safe. The only exception is patients with kidney failure, in whom the dose must be restricted. I especially like magnesium in a powdered form. Taken at night, it provides relaxation and prevents nocturnal leg cramps.

Children under 5 need 200 mg of magnesium a day. Older children and adults need at least 400 mg a day. Sweating during sports requires more magnesium, and doses up to 1,000 mg a day are helpful.

Chromium

Chromium is a trace mineral that helps insulin lower blood sugar in diabetics and also prevents hypoglycemic reactions.

Found mainly in meats and whole grains, this mineral reduces the dose of glucose-lowering medications needed by Type 2 diabetics. Along with niacin and certain amino acids, chromium forms glucose tolerance factor (GTF), a molecule that enhances insulin action by helping insulin bind to cellular membranes. Insulin cannot work until it links to cell membranes, so chromium serves an essential function in assisting the action of insulin. Chromium deficiency may result from eating processed foods, and crops grown in soil depleted of minerals may also be chromium deficient.

Some controversy has been generated about the possibility of chromium toxicity. However, in the recommended adult dose of up to 1000 micrograms (one mg), no side effects have been reported. In fact, it takes 3000 times the adult dose for any side effects to occur. While chromosome changes were found in hamster ovarian cells at that dosage level, other animal studies found no chromium toxicity in any concentration. With this in mind, I feel confident recommending the following dosages for diabetics:

- Under age 6, 100 mcg per day
- 6 to 12, 200 mcg per day
- 13 and over, 600 up to a maximum of 1,000 mcg (1 mg) per day

Vanadium

Many studies support the use of vanadium in blood-sugar control. This trace mineral is ingested in microgram amounts in the normal diet (a microgram is a millionth of a gram, or one thirty-millionth of an ounce). Taken in larger doses, it strengthens the effect of insulin. The usual compound, vanadyl sulfate, helps normalize the blood sugar level, thereby permitting a substantial reduction of insulin dose. It also has a beneficial effect on cholesterol levels and blood pressure, causing both to decline. Side effects are unusual and involve only mild gastrointestinal irritation. I recommend the following dosages for diabetics:

- Under age 6, 5 mg per day
- 6 to 12, 10 mg per day

- 13 and over, 20 mg per day
- Adults, 50 mg per day

B Vitamins

Among many other adverse effects, deficiencies of B vitamins, especially thiamin, biotin, and pyridoxine, result in reduced glucose tolerance and make it more difficult to control diabetes. Thiamin is a crucial factor in maintaining cardiac and neurologic function. Biotin maintains healthy skin, hair, and nails. Pyridoxine is used to treat anemia and prevent seizures. Vitamin B_{12}, deficient more often in diabetics, maintains cognitive and neurologic function and prevents anemia. The minimum daily requirement of B vitamins should be taken in a daily supplement and higher doses employed to treat cardiac and neurologic disorders.

Gymnema Sylvestre

A number of different herbs have been used effectively in treating diabetes. Onions, garlic, bitter melon, holy basil, fenugreek, salt bush, pterocarpus, ginseng, and banaba all have documented efficacy in lowering blood sugar by increasing the action of insulin. The one I use most often is called gymnema sylvestre. It is a plant found in the forests of India. It has no side effects and does not cause hypoglycemia. The usual dose is 200 mg a day in children and 400 mg in adults.

GINSENG REDUCES BLOOD SUGAR

A study published in the journal *Archives of Internal Medicine* (Vol. 160, No. 7, April 10, 2000) shows that American ginseng reduces blood sugar. The authors, from St. Michael's Hospital and the University of Toronto, said they found taking ginseng before a meal reduces blood sugar in people with and without diabetes. Lead investigator Dr. Vladimir Vuksan said the findings may have important implications for the treatment and prevention of diabetes. "Although preliminary, these findings are encouraging and indicate that American ginseng's potential role in diabetes should be taken seriously and investigated further," Vuksan said. "Controlling after-meal blood sugar levels is a very important strategy in managing diabetes. It may also be important in the prevention of diabetes in those who have not yet developed the disease.

Essential Fatty Acids

There are good fats and bad fats. Bad fats are the ones that raise cholesterol and cause arteriosclerosis, gall bladder disease, obesity, and other health problems. The good fats are the ones the body requires to exist. These are called essential fatty acids. They must be obtained from food because the body is not able to manufacture them. They constitute parts of cell membranes and are used to make hormones. Essential fats are of two kinds, omega-3 and omega-6 fatty acids. Omega-3 fatty acids are made by plants, especially microscopic algae. Fish eat these algae and store the omega-3 fatty acids in their tissues. Coldwater fish, especially salmon, tuna, mackerel, and sardines, have the highest content. Omega-3 fatty acids are also plentiful in some vegetable oils, especially flaxseed and hemp oils.

Once you ingest omega-3 fatty acids, your body converts them to docosahexaenoic acid (DHA) and eicosapentaenoic acid (EPA). DHA is highly concentrated in the brain and is critical for proper neurologic function. When the brain is deficient in DHA, our ability to learn suffers and we may become depressed. EPA, on the other hand, forms prostaglandins and leucotrienes, hormones that affect immune function, inflammatory responses, and blood coagulation.

Omega-3 fatty acids improve blood-sugar control in diabetics and have a number of other benefits. They are used to treat inflammatory bowel disease, skin inflammations, multiple sclerosis, allergic conditions, and some forms of kidney disease.

Omega-6 fatty acids are found in beans, nuts, seeds, and grains. They also comprise cell membranes and produce prostaglandins and other hormones. Deficiencies of omega-6 fatty acids cause thinning or loss of hair, skin rashes such as eczema, behavioral problems, and growth impairment. Essential fatty acids reduce the risk of heart disease. Eating one fish meal a week reduces the risk of lethal arrhythmia by 40 percent. Fish oils lower blood pressure, lower triglycerides, and maintain the potency of cardiac bypass grafts. They also lower blood sugar by enhancing insulin activity.

A diet rich in essential fatty acids prolongs life by lowering the risk of heart disease. Case in point: the Mediterranean and Eskimo diets are both high in foods containing omega-3 and omega-6 fatty acids. They have very high fat diets, but a very low incidence of heart disease. In Crete, an island near Greece, fat comprises 40 percent of caloric intake, yet the mortality rate from heart disease is only one twentieth the rate in the United States. Clearly it is the type of fats we eat, not the amount, that is responsible for adverse health consequences.

The recommended dose of omega-3 and omega-6 fatty acids is estimated to be at least 3 grams a day. An excellent source of essential fatty acids is flaxseed oil, containing both omega-3 and omega-6 fatty acids. It must be refrigerated and can't be used for cooking, as heat degrades it. It can be added to yogurt, salads, and protein drinks, or mixed with peanut or almond butter and spread on bread. One tablespoon of flaxseed oil provides 2.2 grams of omega-6 fatty acids and 7.7 grams of omega-3 fatty acids. One tablespoon a day is sufficient for diabetic children 12 years old or younger. Older diabetic children should take two tablespoons a day.

Once we put young people on a program of nutritional supplements, their diabetes becomes much better controlled. Here is Justin's story:

Justin's Story

Justin was 17 years old when he came to our clinic in April 1997. Four weeks previously, he had developed increasing thirst and urination, fatigue, leg cramps, and a weight loss of 10 pounds. His blood sugar was 970 (ten times normal). Justin's physician diagnosed him as having Type 1 diabetes and treated him with intravenous fluids and insulin. He ate a 3,200-calorie, high-carbohydrate diet. His insulin dose in the morning was 18 units of long-acting and 5 units of regular insulin. Before dinner, he took 12 units of long-acting and 5 units of regular insulin, a total of 40 units of insulin a day. His parents modified his diet so that it was high in protein, whole grains, salad, and fruit. His C-peptide level, a measure of his body's natural insulin production, was reduced at 0.9. His fructosamine level, an indicator of blood-sugar control, was elevated at 339 (normal is less than 268).

Justin was placed on the program we prescribe at the clinic— a diet composed of low-glycemic-index foods, a regimen of nutritional supplements, and daily exercise. After consulting with our nutritionist, the French toast, pancakes, syrup, and orange juice he had for breakfast, as well as the ham, mayonnaise, yogurt, bananas, and orange juice he had for lunch were eliminated. The bread, rolls, and potato chips he ate with dinner also went by the wayside. Instead he was placed on a diet of low-glycemic-index foods, high in protein, without bread, cereals, and other refined carbohydrates, without dairy products or juices. His main foods were vegetables, whole grains, some fruits, nuts and seeds, fish, chicken, and specified meats.

Justin was also placed on a nutritional supplement program, which included:

- Multivitamins, 10 tablets
- Magnesium-potassium capsules, 4
- An omega-3 and -6 fatty acid preparation, 2 tablets
- A combination of sprouted grain extracts, 2 teaspoons
- Trace minerals, 1 teaspoon
- Water, filtered or distilled, ten 8-ounce glasses
- Niacinamide, 3 grams
- Ginkgo, 180 milligrams
- Biotin, 16 milligrams
- Vanadyl sulfate, 150 milligrams
- Lipoic acid, 600 milligrams
- Coenzyme Q10, 200 milligrams
- Magnesium, chelated, 600 milligrams

Like Grant and other diabetic patients we saw during this period, Justin was also started on 20 milligrams a day of Muraglycine.

Justin's parents were amazed at the changes in his health after just one week on this program. His fasting blood sugar fell to a level of 90–105, well within the normal range of 70–110 and most surprising of all to his family, he was able to discontinue insulin.

For two years, Justin remained on this program and did very well without taking any supplemental insulin. In July 1998, his fasting blood-sugar level was 113 and glycohemoglobin 7.2, demonstrating excellent control of his blood sugar. Ultimately he had to stop using Muraglycine because of financial considerations, and at that point was started back on insulin.

It is remarkable that Justin was able to remain completely off insulin for a duration far beyond the honeymoon period normally experienced, with excellent blood-sugar control. His story reveals the dramatic and rapid changes that can occur in juvenile diabetics when they are put on our program. For periods of time ranging from months to years, many experience good blood-sugar control even to the point of discontinuing insulin.

I am not trying to suggest that juvenile diabetics can be treated without insulin, but rather to indicate that lifestyle changes coupled with potent nutritional supplementation can substantially reduce the dose of insulin and support good diabetic control. Therefore I advocate the following:

- Appropriate nutritional supplements that can reduce the dose of insulin required, improving blood-sugar control.
- Supplements that allow the body to get the most mileage out of the natural insulin the beta cells still produce.
- Supplements that prevent, limit, and perhaps even reverse the vascular and organ damage seen in diabetics.

Remember: the lower the dose of insulin, the lower the frequency and severity of hypogylcemic episodes.

CHAPTER 8

Parents and Children:
Partners in Healing

Brian's Story

Several months before his first visit to my office, Brian developed a respiratory illness that lasted six weeks. Shortly thereafter, he began having symptoms of unusual thirst, high urinary frequency, and weight loss. His blood-sugar level was measured at 694 (70 to 110 is normal).

Brian was diagnosed by his physician as having Type 1 diabetes, a development that often follows an apparent viral infection in children, perhaps due to antibodies against the virus that cross-react with pancreatic cells. The doctor recommended that Brian should begin ongoing insulin therapy.

But because Brian's parents had read about natural therapies for controlling diabetes, they refused insulin therapy and started him on a rigorous diet that consisted of beans, pasta, Basmati rice and brown rice, vegetables, chicken, and small quantities of fruit. He began to take vanadyl sulfate (a trace mineral that enhances insulin activity), biotin (a B vitamin that helps control blood sugar), magnesium, and potassium supplements. His blood sugar fell to 240, down from 694 but still more than twice what it should be.

Brian first came to our clinic in March 1996. He was 4 feet 11 inches tall, weighed 75 pounds, and looked healthy. His initial lab tests showed that his blood-sugar level was 163, and his glycohemoglobin (a measurement of average blood-sugar control) was high at 9.5 (a superior level is less than 7). His cholesterol profile was normal. His C-peptide level (a measure of insulin production, normally between 2 and 4) was 0.87, indicating that some of his pancreatic beta cells were still producing insulin, but at a reduced rate.

I started Brian on a daily exercise program and changed his diet to include a higher intake of complex carbohydrates, emphasizing whole grains and more protein. This was done because complex carbohydrates and protein generally cause only modest blood-sugar elevations after eating, thus requiring less insulin to control the blood sugar. Meat and dairy products were eliminated from his diet, though he did continue to eat chicken and fish. Brian also received a broad-spectrum vitamin and mineral regimen, along with targeted nutritional supplements intended for the management of his diabetes.

Over the next two months, although Brian felt well, his blood-sugar levels were in the 200 range and he lost an additional 2 pounds. We discussed his situation and decided he would be best served by starting insulin therapy. He began taking Humulin insulin 70/30, which is predominantly a long-acting insulin with a small amount of rapid-acting insulin. With 3 units in the morning and 3 units before dinner, his morning blood sugars were 94–115, and evening blood sugars about 150. He gained 3 pounds and grew an inch.

In March 1999, three years after his first visit to our clinic, 15-year-old Brian was 5 feet 5 inches and weighed 108 pounds. He had had only one infection in the prior year. Academically excellent, he was first in his class of 93 students. He exercised, with pushups and rollerblading.

Brian was taking a mixture of short- and long-acting insulin three times a day. Hypoglycemic reactions occurred once a month and were mild. He took his supplements regularly.

Like many diabetics, after the diagnosis of diabetes had been made, Brian experienced a "honeymoon" period, during which the pancreas recovered some of its ability to make insulin. For quite a while he was able to avoid the use of insulin entirely. Even eight months after the onset of diabetes, his blood sugar was controlled with a small dose of only 6 units of insulin daily. The supplements permitted a lower dose of insulin, softening the peaks and valleys of blood-sugar fluctuation.

We often see that the honeymoon period is prolonged with the right diet and specific nutritional supplements, which in addition to reducing insulin requirements, also seem to reduce the stress on the pancreas to produce more insulin. During the honeymoon period, the pancreas, for unknown reasons, reasserts its ability to produce insulin. This period can be extended by such measures as diet, exercise, and supplements, which prevent blood-sugar elevations and thereby reduce the requirement for insulin. One supplement that is useful at this time is the B vitamin niacinamide. There is experimental evidence that niacinamide may lessen or slow down pancreatic damage when given early in the course of Type 1 diabetes.

Eventually, however, Brian's pancreas gave out, and higher doses of insulin were needed. At that point, he could simply have taken the insulin and skipped the rest of the program, but he chose to stay on it. Without this program of diet, supplements, and exercise, it is unlikely that Brian would have been able to achieve such excellent control of his blood sugar. I also believe that antioxidant supplementation over the years will ultimately help to prevent damage to his eyes, kidneys, and cardiovascular system. Beyond this, Brian has gained the confidence of knowing how to control his illness. In the long run, his understanding and knowledge will allow for continued good blood-sugar control under changing circumstances. In short, he will be able to adjust.

Brian continues to thrive, both physically and intellectually. His parents, who were initially very worried about his health and his future, are extremely pleased with his progress.

As a board-certified internist with many years of experience treating diabetes as well as a multitude of other medical conditions, I have seen how difficult it can be living with a medical problem. As a married father with three sons, I have experienced the stress that can be caused by a child's illness. Education, knowing what to expect and how to resolve problems, is essential in dealing with diabetics, because so much is known about how to keep this disease from progressing.

Only in the last decade has it been proven that controlling blood sugar prevents diabetic complications. A landmark paper, published in 1993, demonstrated that tight diabetic control reduced the onset of eye complications by 76 percent and the progression of eye disease by 54 percent, compared with patients treated less vigorously (The Diabetics Control and Complications Trial Research Group: "The Effect of Intensive Treatment of Diabetes on the Development and Progression of Long-Term Complications in Insulin-Dependent Diabetes Mellitus;" *New Eng. J. Med.* 1993; 329: 977–86). The risk of kidney disease was reduced by 54 percent and neuropathy by 60 percent. Another study showed similar benefits from tight control of Type 2 diabetes (UK Prospective Diabetes Study Group: "Intensive Blood Glucose Control with Sulfonylureas or Insulin Compared with Conventional Treatment and the Risk of Complications in Patients with Type 2 Diabetes;" *The Lancet* 1998; 352: 837-53). In this study, close control of blood sugar offered a 25 percent reduction in eye, kidney, and nerve damage, and a 16 percent reduction in heart attacks.

The major risk of tight control is an increased incidence of hypoglycemia. Following the program offered in this book can lessen this risk by reducing the need for insulin and offering foods that lessen fluctuations in blood sugar.

I wrote this book as a result of my experience in treating diabetic children. Nutritional therapy has been the main approach. Parents came with their children from many states, even though their children were already seeing other physicians for diabetic care. The parents were worried and sometimes confused by conflicting information. They had received inadequate explanations. Some had been given dismal prognoses for their children's health and were very anxious about the future.

I was struck by the fact that in spite of active medical and nutritional attention, the children had diets that were almost uniformly improper and inadequate. They arrived at the clinic snacking on cold cereals or drinking fruit juices and diet soft drinks. The parents were intelligent and conscientious, yet didn't know the difference between simple and complex carbohydrates. They weren't aware of the glycemic index and didn't know how to use nutritional supplements. What they did know was that they needed to know more, and that they would go anywhere necessary to learn it.

I had already seen how many adult diabetics dramatically improved when they learned about nutrition, added specific supplements, and committed themselves to making necessary lifestyle changes. Time after time I saw their blood sugars come under control so that they could reduce their medications or even eliminate them entirely.

Children can do even better, and parents can learn enough to feel secure in managing their children's diabetes.

Parents' Questions About Getting Well

Q. How often should our child see a doctor?
A. Your child should see a physician regularly, usually at three-month intervals. The eyes should be evaluated yearly. Tests of kidney function should be performed at least yearly.

Q. Must the rest of the family eat like this, too?
A. The diet that is healthy for a diabetic is also healthy for the rest of the family. All the members of your family will be healthier if they avoid refined sugars, snack foods and junk foods, additives, and preservatives.

Q. How long should our child take nutritional supplements?
A. One should continue to take them throughout one's lifetime. They will help to prevent complications and keep the blood sugar under better control.

Q. Why did the other doctor tell us not to worry about what our child eats, just to take enough insulin to control the blood sugar?
A. Studies indicate that if the blood sugar is controlled, diabetic complications are greatly reduced. It is a narrow view, however, to believe that blood-sugar control is the only objective. Proper food choices are even more important for diabetic children than other children. They need more nutrients, more fiber, more essential fatty acids. Giving them fast foods, snack foods, salt, and refined foods deprives them of nutrients and sets them up for the same problems of eventual obesity, hypertension, cardiovascular disease, and cancer that the rest of the population faces. Eating low-glycemic-index foods, whole foods, and organic foods helps to prevent these problems. It also makes it easier to regulate glucose levels.

Q. *What if my doctor disagrees with the program you recommend?*
A. It is unlikely your doctor will disapprove. There is no risk, and the value of the program is substantiated in the medical literature. Nevertheless, if your doctor won't support the program, it would be best to find another physician. There's no use having a physician who opposes your plan for your child's health.

Q. *What if our child refuses to cooperate, won't eat the right foods, and keeps looking for fast foods and goodies?*
A. Don't despair. Keep reinforcing the program and offer a proper diet at home. Don't eat bad foods yourself. Set a good example. Compromise. Let your child have some of the foods he or she wants, even if they are undesirable. Over time, with your continued efforts and encouragement, your child will gradually adjust and will very likely come to prefer the taste of good food.

Q. *Is it possible for our child to have a long, healthy life?*
A. Yes. Many diabetics have few medical problems even after decades of dealing with their illness. Proper nutrition, supplements, exercising, and staying thin go a long way toward preventing problems. Improvements in therapy occur every year.

Pharmaceutical Advances in Controlling Diabetes

Over the last decade, there have been a number of pharmaceutical breakthroughs in treating diabetes. Today there are newer and more effective types of insulin, and newer and more powerful oral medications for lowering blood sugar.

These advances are welcome. It will be great to have a new insulin that lasts 24 hours, and an insulin given intranasally (through a nose spray) so that injections won't be necessary. Pancreas transplants are a valuable option in some situations. It will be a relief to monitor blood sugars with a device that reads glucose levels through the skin without need of a needle puncture.

Yet it is a mistake to emphasize pharmaceutical and technological advances at the expense of other holistic approaches to controlling diabetes that are safer and simpler. For example, the traditional approach to treating Type 2 diabetes is to prescribe drugs that actually further increase the production of insulin by the pancreas. This paradoxical approach has been used for over 30 years. It makes no sense to increase insulin levels when insulin levels are already high in Type 2 diabetics.

Recently however, newer medications have been introduced to counter insulin resistance, the real problem in Type 2 diabetes. But even though these drugs may be accompanied by serious side effects like liver damage and even death, many physicians turn to these drugs immediately. Unless the diabetic is already on an adequate program to counter insulin resistance with natural methods like weight loss, exercise, proper food choices, and nutritional supplements, such action is premature and even dangerous.

Reports in medical journals and in popular magazines and newspapers confirm what I see in my practice every day. People both young and old are getting heavier. They are exercising less, traveling more, eating out more frequently in restaurants. A third of the population is obese, and the number is rising. As a result there is also more Type 2 diabetes (even in children) as well as more stress, hypertension, cardiovascular disease, and cancer.

The answer to these problems does not come in a pill bottle or an injection. The answer lies in aggressive lifestyle intervention, focused foremost on nutrition but with the knowledge that exercise, applied supplementation, and a positive attitude are also indispensable. This strategy will prevent obesity and Type 2 diabetes and also help reverse these diseases after they occur. Though we cannot reverse Type 1 diabetes, we can manage it to avoid its complications.

Helping Kids to Make Wise Food Choices

For many parents, the most trying part of educating their diabetic children lies in helping them understand why they can't eat certain foods or behave in certain ways. Because they are so worried, they sometimes fall into the role of food dictator, telling their children that they can't have this or that because it will either make them gain weight or wreak havoc with blood sugars. If you've ever tried this approach, you already know that being a food cop doesn't help to establish a successful obesity or diabetes management program. Persistent denial does not encourage compliance; instead, it creates frustration and animosity. Children need to understand why certain foods are better for them than others, and they also need to learn from parents who set an example with their own healthy eating habits. When children make choices that are best for their health, they need this smart behavior reinforced. This is where your creativity, insight into what your own child likes, and your own sense of play come in. Figure out what's meaningful to your child in terms of games and make getting well through adopting wise eating and exercise habits an enjoyable experience. Start cooking with your children. Find recipes for tasty alternatives to prohibited dishes, such as desserts. The magic of transforming raw ingredients into delicious treats can be a great incentive for children, upping their interest in healthy nutrition!

No matter how anxious or exasperated you become, don't turn into a prohibitionist. Stay in good humor. Dietary peccadilloes are not fatal mistakes. You can joke about them, maintain a positive attitude, and guide your children to make better choices in the future.

Using Nutritional Supplements

Certain nutrients offer particular benefits to diabetics and represent an essential part of the program. These nutrients include essential fatty acids, B vitamins, antioxidant vitamins C and E, magnesium, coenzyme Q10, lipoic acid, chromium, and vanadium. Adding them to a diabetic's diet, along with exercise, stress reduction, and dietary changes, can make a radical difference in a diabetic's health.

Incorporating Exercise

Because exercise reduces the need for insulin, it's probably the most important element in a diabetic's program for health. Introduce your children to a variety of sports when they are young, and encourage them to choose the one they like. Stress the importance of physical activity for good diabetes control, and encourage children to exercise daily. Make exercise and sports a regular part of family life.

REINFORCING HEALTHY DECISIONS

Create rewards for making good decisions. For example, you could set a 25-cent reward for each time your children have fruit instead of ice cream. Or, if you'd rather not use money as an incentive, consider awarding points for good eating habits and time spent exercising. Work out a system together that equates accomplishments with a point system, and then decide how many points are required to realize various rewards.

Encourage Your Kids to Share Their Feelings

Talk to your children about how having diabetes and dealing with restrictions and lifestyle changes is making them feel. Because suppressed resentment only leads to more resistance, encourage youngsters to express their emotions. When things don't go well, help your children put yesterday behind them. Make sure they know you are on their side—that you are there to help them succeed.

Make success a game. Chart your children's progress in bright colors on large cardboard sheets. Use graphs or stickers. Put a quarter in a jar for every balanced meal. Let your children spend the money on their choices at the end of each week.

Children aren't famous for their patience, so don't make them wait too long for their rewards. Make what they've earned really special by inviting a friend or creating special events, holidays, and birthday parties.

Work with your children to produce homemade books on nutrition, with photographs, cutout illustrations, and recipes, as well as their impressions and opinions about living with diabetes.

This approach will make your children feel loved. In the end, this is the most important message.

A Child's Health Crisis Can Draw the Family Closer

A child's illness can make the family unit closer or cause it to disintegrate. Your aim should be to give the family an opportunity to reassess itself and to evaluate how the family dynamic must change in order to put the necessary energy into helping the diabetic child get well without overlooking the needs of other children and adults in the family. Modern life is hectic, and parents feel swamped by too many responsibilities. The pressure is increased when both parents work outside the home and/or care for ailing parents. Those who are separated, divorced and living apart while sharing child-care responsibilities have even more agonizing issues.

Managing diabetes when the diabetic child belongs to two different families can seem confusing and even overwhelming. Because your child's health is at a critical passage, this is a time to make great efforts to overlook the bitterness and differences that led to separation and divorce. What you must really focus on is your child's well-being and his relationship with each parent. Is this relationship nurturing and meaningful? Is it a source of strength and rejuvenation for both parents and children? If the relationship is weak on one side, it will almost certainly be weak on the other. What can be done to improve the dynamic of these relationships so that the child feels less stressed and more valued? What can be done to improve communication between parents who live in different households so that keeping the diabetes in good control is easier? Both parents need to understand and agree on the management plan. If the parents disagree, the child will receive conflicting messages, and it will not be possible to establish consistency. The child may become confused and angry.

A child's illness forces the family to confront such issues with commitment, passion, honesty, and friendship—qualities often ignored in the superficial rush of daily life. Being strong enough to put your wounded feelings aside in order to help your ailing child may well be the most heroic act of your lifetime. The harder the struggle, the greater the significance and the more profound and enduring the relationship.

Developing Good Health Habits

Encourage proper chewing

When a child has diabetes, things once taken for granted in childhood assume greater importance. Like thorough chewing of food. To improve digestion and encourage weight control, encourage your children to eat slowly and chew their food well. Carbohydrate digestion begins in the mouth. The amylase enzyme present in saliva is an important component in this first stage of digestion. Thoroughly chewing grains and other complex carbohydrates prepares the food to yield the nutrients that our bodies need. Each bite of food should be chewed until it is completely saturated with saliva. In this way, the full nutritional value of the food will be released. Inadequate chewing of carbohydrates or washing food down with excessive liquids causes a heavy feeling and can result in bloating, gas, or pain. Thorough chewing also gives the stomach enough time to feel full, so that the child doesn't eat more than is actually needed. All family members can benefit from this advice.

Get plenty of sleep

Sleep deprivation causes impairment of metabolic activities and may promote the onset of diseases like diabetes, hypertension, brain dysfunction, and immune disorders. Few of us actually get as much sleep as we need, especially children. In the last 90 years, the average adult has lost 1.5 hours of sleep. In 1910, an average night's sleep lasted 9 hours. Now it lasts only 7.5 hours. It seems we now have other priorities.

Sleep deprivation adversely affects body functions. In a study documenting the metabolic changes associated with loss of sleep ("Impact of Sleep Debt on Metabolic and Endocrine Function," Spiegel, K., et al, *The Lancet;* Volume 354; Oct. 23, 1999), healthy young men were allowed only 4 hours of sleep a night. After one week the following changes were seen:

- Their blood-sugar levels rose, and they produced more insulin. As a result, they developed an insulin-resistant state, similar to that of Type 2 diabetes.
- Their adrenal cortisol production was increased, which suppresses immune function and impairs memory and learning ability.
- Their thyroid hormone levels were increased.
- Their sympathetic nervous system activity increased over their parasympathetic activity, an imbalance that adversely affects blood pressure, cardiac activity, and kidney function.

Getting needed sleep will benefit not only the brain but also coordination, concentration, mood, and alertness. To be sure that kids get sufficient time to sleep, dream, and nurture the body, try to get them to bed at a reasonable hour every night. Keep sleepovers to a minimum. Avoid scary movies, sweet foods, and caffeine-containing drinks before bedtime. Read to them before bed. To calm them and set the stage for sleep, give children a teaspoon of calcium-magnesium powder in water just before bed.

28 Tips for Keeping Your Child Healthy

Use the following checklist to examine your family lifestyle in order to evaluate what you've achieved and what areas still need work.

1. Ensure a proper diet, emphasizing whole foods and avoiding processed foods.

The foods you see most advertised are often the least good for you and your children, especially diabetic children. That's particularly true of fast foods, snack foods, cold cereals, donuts, cakes and ice cream, all foods that can just be picked up, poured out and eaten because they need no preparation. Such foods are appealing because shopping and meal preparation take a lot of time, and it's often easier to turn to convenience foods and fast foods when both parents are working. Driving to a restaurant or opening a package can be mighty attractive when you're exhausted, the kids are cranky, and the idea of giving them foods that appeal to their taste buds because they're sweet, salty, and crunchy seems an easy way to make everyone happy. But that type of answer can have long-term consequences.

We are in a dangerous spot. If we do not change, we are in for a difficult time.

But there is time for change. A whole lifetime.

Get the right information on what to eat, how to find it, and how to prepare it. The next chapter of this book contains instructions on meal planning and preparation. There are also directions on how to find more information and where to buy food.

It is not true that good diets are too restrictive. After all, processed and fast foods are fairly new arrivals. People lived without them for many centuries. All vegetables, most fruits, nuts, seeds, beans, lentils, fish, chicken, meat, eggs, many grains, and some dairy products are appropriate for diabetics and others who want to lose weight and lead a healthier life. There is plenty of variety.

THE PRINCIPLES OF GOOD NUTRITION

Knowing what to buy and what to feed your diabetic child and your family isn't difficult if you follow these guidelines:

- Obtain fresh, whole foods. Wash produce thoroughly, especially if it isn't organic.
- Buy organic. These foods are better since they are richer in nutrients and free of herbicides, pesticides, hormones, and antibiotics, which can be harmful to every member of your family.
- Avoid processed foods like snack foods and junk foods because they are nutrient-poor and low in fiber. These also have had anti-nutrients added to them, such as trans-fatty acids, which interfere with

the utilization of beneficial omega-3 and omega-6 fatty acids.

- Buy grains closest in form to whole grains, avoiding those that have been milled and pulverized into breads and pastas while being emptied of fiber, vitamins, and minerals.
- Serve fruits, not fruit juices.
- Make water, not soft drinks or lemonade, the beverage of choice.
- Avoid refined sugar.
- Investigate anything that comes wrapped before you buy it. Learn the meanings of the words listed under food contents.
- Serve more vegetables, especially those organically grown. Present them raw or steamed, and in combination with other vegetables.
- Buy free-range chickens and eggs.
- Be sure your meat doesn't come from abused, malnourished, and toxin-laden animals.
- Skip meat by-products, like sandwich meats, that contain nitrates.
- Select fresh fish whenever possible.
- Prepare meals that have variety.
- Eat at home whenever possible, rather than at restaurants.
- Enlist children's help with shopping, meal preparation, and cleanup.

When parents and other children in the family follow the same rules required for diabetic or obese children, they will be healthier and live longer.

2. Ignore false information.

Though this sounds difficult, it's easier than you think. Realize that big business will not protect your or your children's health. In order to survive, business must place morality second to income. It will offer biased information, influence politicians, and invade schools, ballparks, television, and magazines with advertising. It will dissemble. It will lie. It will use clever copy writing and persuasive athletes to establish poor eating habits.

3. Introduce change slowly.

Decide which changes are most important and easiest to incorporate into your family's lifestyle. Explain things to your child and give him time to adjust, to realize there are satisfactory replacements for foods he should not be eating.

Try to get agreement on making improvements. The program works well only when everyone, including other family members, buys into it.

Don't feel that you have to change your child's whole world overnight. It is better to make gradual corrections than to insist that everything be done perfectly at once.

4. Educate yourself, educate others.

The nutritional recommendations in this book are not arbitrary but based on excellent, validated medical research performed over decades. As you read this research, you will be impressed by its implications for health and well-being. The more you study and the more you know, the easier it will be to distinguish what is true from what is not, and to create a healthier situation for your diabetic or obese child and for all the other members of your family.

Information alone does not always resolve problems. When dealing with lifestyle changes, it is also necessary to undo the dependency on prior types of behavior. For example, there are millions of people who believe that cigarettes are bad for their health but are still unable to stop smoking. Still, it is better to know, and then to work to make the right things happen.

Family members should meet together, to discuss what needs to be done to help a diabetic or obese child. Parents should read books together with their children on subjects including diabetes, nutrition, pollution, and other subjects impacting health.

5. Find a good physician.

You need more than a physician with good training and experience. The best doctor to treat your diabetic child is one with whom you can establish rapport and trust and who can communicate effectively with you and with your child. The ideal physician is not one who decides for you, but one who provides you with information and guidance in making and implementing your own decisions. After all, the responsibility for health decisions rests not with the physician, but with the patient and the patient's family. To assign it elsewhere ignores the reality that it is the patient, not the physician, who must bear the consequences. Each patient is different. Physicians cannot use their own knowledge and judgment to substitute for their patients' understanding. If physicians put their own preferences in place of the patient's goals, there will be resistance and little positive movement. Even in the case of little children, education should start at the very beginning of treatment, by conveying simple ideas and advancing to more complicated ones as the child attains more understanding and greater maturity.

You need a physician who can communicate, answer questions, and be patient with your upsets and failures. Your physician must be accessible as a human being as well as a professional.

6. Give your child vitamin and mineral supplements.

Nutritional deficiencies exist even in this land of plenty, not because of starvation but because we eat the wrong foods. For example, few people eat the recommended number of five servings of vegetables and fruits a day, resulting in deficiencies of fiber and magnesium. Trace metals such as zinc, copper, selenium, manganese, and molybdenum may also be deficient, partly because of depleted agricultural soils. Selenium deficiency in particular has been causally related to several cancers and heart failure.

Diabetes causes substantial loss of nutrients in the urine, and deficiencies may cause further elevations of blood sugar as well as worsen potential complications. Particular care is therefore needed to ensure that diabetic children receive daily supplements.

Certain nutrients should be provided in greater than usual amounts, because of their special benefits, and given at meal times. Vitamin C, vitamin E, coenzyme Q10, and lipoic acid have strong antioxidant effects and preserve tissue integrity. Magnesium, essential fatty acids, lipoic acid, several of the B vitamins, chromium, and vanadium enhance the action of insulin. In Type 1 diabetes, they reduce the necessary dose of insulin. In Type 2 diabetes, they may wholly eliminate the need for diabetic medications. Gymnema sylvestre is an herb that also increases insulin activity. Recommended doses for all of these supplements are listed in chapter 7.

It is an error to exclude nutritional supplementation from the care of any diabetic, or for that matter from any adult or child, even those in good health.

7. Eat at home.

Most restaurants do not serve organic foods, sprouted-grain breads, or filtered water. They do serve meals loaded with salt and sugar, introducing the menu along with lots of bread on the table. The temptation to have soft drinks and desserts is high in restaurants. Fried foods are frequently on the menu, especially in fast-food restaurants. The oils used in frying may be old and rancid and contain dangerous trans-fatty acids, leading to accelerated atherosclerosis.

If you go out to eat, choose restaurants that offer superior fare. Often these are health-food restaurants, but other restaurants may provide good fresh foods without a lot of added oils. When ordering salads, use only vinegar and virgin olive oil, and add them yourself so you can use less. Do not order the soft drinks or desserts.

Of course it is hard for parents to make and serve three meals and snacks every day. Kitchen burnout is always a threat. But other family members, like spouses and older children, should provide regular assistance with shopping, cooking, and cleaning up. The diabetic child, in particular, should be involved with meal planning and preparation.

8. Have meals together.

The family meal is a great opportunity for bonding. It is also a great time to reinforce healthy eating habits. A large Harvard study (published in the *Archives of Family Medicine,* May 2000) shows that children who frequently eat with their parents have healthier eating habits than those who rarely do. The study found that children who had family meals were one and a half times as likely to eat five servings of fruits and vegetables every day as those who rarely ate with their parents. A nutritional analysis of the diets showed that children who frequently ate with their parents had the highest intake of such important nutrients as calcium, fiber, folate, iron, and vitamins B and E. The study also found that children who ate family dinners often tended to have healthier diets throughout the day.

9. Promote daily sports and exercise.

Plan ahead to do physical activities like skiing, hiking, or boating together as a family. Take vacations that involve a lot of sporting activities. The more your children are involved in sports when they are young, the more they will pursue sports when they get older.

10. Use filtered or bottled water.

11. Take care of your child's teeth.

12. Travel with your child.

13. Watch television rarely.

14. Make sure your child gets plenty of rest.

15. Spend time with your child.

16. Make time for your child.

17. Set a good example for your child in terms of eating well.

18. Support your child's interests and ambitions.

19. Compliment your child.

20. Keep criticism positive.

21. Lower stress by keeping parental problems private. Play games and pursue hobbies with your child.

22. Choose humorous, upbeat, or inspiring movies for your children.

Violent or scary movies can make it difficult for them to sleep, and losing sleep can be harmful to diabetics.

23. Encourage reading.

24. Encourage music and art.

25. Encourage laughter.

26. Encourage singing.

27. Love your child.

28. Become an activist lobbying for good nutrition.

Because politics and health are unavoidably entwined, work with other parents to persuade legislators that children should be offered healthy meals in the lunchroom and educated about proper nutrition in the classroom. Take your cue from Mothers Against Drunk Driving, an organization composed of volunteers who have mastered working in the political arena to change the attitudes of people and politicians. They have changed laws and saved lives.

Your child's health can turn around just like a little girl named Jackie, whom we treated at our clinic.

Jackie's Story

For weeks, 10-year-old Jackie had been feeling unusually tired and had developed a respiratory infection for which she was being treated with steroids because of wheezing. When her weakness increased, she was taken to the emergency room, where doctors discovered her blood sugar was extremely high, accompanied by an imbalance of her acid-base status. She was diagnosed with juvenile diabetes, admitted to the intensive care unit, and was observed to be lethargic. A radiological procedure revealed swelling of her brain, a serious condition caused by her markedly elevated glucose level.

A physician in the intensive care unit told Jackie's mother that when children die from diabetes, they usually die because of brain swelling. That night was a long and scary one for Jackie's mother.

The next day Jackie started to improve. The brain swelling resolved. She became increasingly alert and was discharged after five days and put on a low dose of 7 units of insulin a day. During the next six months, her blood sugar remained almost normal. She was much more energetic, although she had two episodes of mild hypoglycemia.

There was a strong family history of diabetes, involving three of her mother's relatives. Her father's sister had developed diabetes as a child, became blind at the age of 25, and died when she was 28. Jackie's parents were justifiably worried about their daughter.

One dietician advised her mother to "just have Jackie eat less." Other advice was to count the grams of carbohydrates she ate and administer insulin accordingly. Jackie's mother said she hated conventional medicine, with its emphasis on a drug for every problem. She brought her daughter to our clinic for a different kind of recommendation.

After three months, Jackie's blood sugar was under good control. She tested her own blood sugars and gave herself her own insulin injections. She was doing home schooling, so there was no concern about school meals. She liked homemade soups and ate organic chicken and low-fat meats.

Jackie rode her bike or walked for an hour every day. She played softball and went to a local gym twice a week. She found exercise effective in keeping her blood sugar down. Because she and her family had learned how to manage diabetes, Jackie felt good and had a positive attitude about herself and her future. She had gained the knowledge and ability to assure continued success.

CHAPTER 9

The Nutritional Program

The following pages offer meal plans and cooking tips that incorporate the ideas and information presented earlier in this book. Diane Lara, the nutritionist with whom I have worked closely for four years, wrote this section. Additional recipes can be found on my web page, *www.allansosinmd.com*.

Helpful Hints

Acid-Alkaline Balance

A proper balance of our daily diet is very important. We can be pretty certain of maintaining this balance if we eat 70 percent alkaline foods (fruits and vegetables) and 30 percent acid foods (meats and grains). Sprouted, flourless breads are alkaline.

Cooking Methods

When cooking food, the best and most healthful method is to steam, poach, broil, bake, or sauté (in broth, not oil or butter). However, a thin film of coconut or olive oil may be used to begin. Keep frying to a minimum using coconut oil. It is a safe, saturated fat not damaged by frying.

Cookware

Aluminum cookware should not be used since the aluminum can leak out into the food. High concentrations of aluminum have been found in the brain tissue of Alzheimer's patients. The best cookware from a health standpoint is stainless steel, glass, or good quality non-stick. (Caution: Abrasive scouring of stainless cookware scratches surfaces releasing toxic metals underneath.)

Foods in Order of Preference

1. Fresh, organic if possible
2. Frozen, unsalted, unsweetened
3. Canned only if necessary

Fruits

Fruits are very important, but the sugar content is much higher than that of vegetables. One or two pieces of fruit are sufficient each day. Also, try to vary the fruits you eat as much as possible. The fruits and vegetables that you eat should be organically grown, if possible. These delicate foods absorb a great deal of the pesticide sprays that are used on them, the worst being strawberries and apples. Therefore, you would be doing yourself and your family a great service by attempting to obtain as many foods as possible from sources that can provide unsprayed produce.

Liquids

Keep liquids to a minimum with meals as they can dilute digestive enzymes, causing loss of nutrients due to food not being properly broken down. However, we all enjoy some beverage with meals, so a little herb tea or some non-icy, pure water may be taken (both icy and very hot liquids interfere with proper digestion). Remember to chew each bite of food until wet with saliva before swallowing.

Meats and Poultry

CAUTION: All animal products are very high in fat! Ask for organic cage-free chicken and turkey, and range-grazed beef. They should be free of chemicals, hormones, and antibiotics. Avoid all preserved meats, i.e., bacon, ham, bologna, pastrami, salami, hot dogs, corned beef, and all lunch meats. These are truly the dregs of the food chain and are loaded with chemicals. Also, avoid all charred and smoked meats and fish (also charred toast); these contain carcinogenic (cancer-causing) substances.

Good Oils

Use oils that are organic and packaged in light-excluding containers, which protect oils from rancidity due to exposure to light (air and heat are not the only culprits). Some good oils are olive, coconut, sesame, safflower, and flaxseed oils.

Bad Oils

Commercial: Polyunsaturated vegetable oils (including most expelled or cold-pressed). All contribute to free-radical damage to healthy cells due to poor processing (margarine, fried food, restaurant oils, etc.)

Packaged Desserts and Sweets: (These Should Be Avoided)

They are loaded with chemical additives and preservatives. The chemicals that are placed in these products are there specifically to allow these items to stay on the market shelf for weeks, months, or even years without molding. These chemicals are called "enzyme inhibitors," and when you eat these products, these same enzyme inhibitors interfere with your own enzyme utilization. Your enzymes are the spark plugs that turn the healthy foods you eat into cell-building material. When you eat desserts loaded with chemicals, you interfere with your own ability to break down food properly. The enzyme inhibitors in the dessert are actually "inhibiting" your enzymes, too. Bake healthy desserts made from whole grains, whole-grain flours, fruits, nuts, brown-rice syrup, xylitol or stevia, and coconut oil or butter as they can withstand high heat.

Proper Storage

Remember that all natural, unprocessed foods should be refrigerated because they are "whole" foods containing all of their natural enzymes and oils, which will rapidly spoil or become rancid at room temperature.

Soft Drinks

Try to avoid these health-robbing drinks. The aluminum cans they are packaged in are toxic. They are full of sugar or artificial sweeteners, and they upset digestion when combined with food. In addition, the acid and carbonation can deplete calcium from our bones as the body attempts to neutralize the acid pH with alkalizing minerals. Many of these drinks contain caffeine where least expected—e.g., orange sodas.

Vegetables

These should be the predominant ingredients in our diets. Five different vegetables should be eaten each day: two cooked and three raw, with seven different vegetables eaten each week.

Water

The water that your family drinks is very important, and tap water is not a healthy choice. Bottled spring water or, preferably, filtered water is much healthier and tastier.

Most Important

When shopping for groceries, read the labels on the foods you are considering. The fewer ingredients in a product, the better, and if you can't understand it—*Don't buy it!*

Reading Labels

The Food and Drug Administration requires that all packaged foods list their ingredients on the label. It has become difficult to purchase high-quality, nutrient-dense foods. Most foods on market shelves are extensively refined, particularly grain-based, pre-packaged foods like breads, cereals, crackers, and baked goods. The milling of grain removes fiber (the bran and the germ), along with essential fatty acids, vitamins, and minerals. All that is left is the starchy white flour used for baking. While quite delicious, white flour is totally lacking in nutrients and creates deficiencies when it replaces other, more nourishing foods. This was revealed in a study done in the 1930s.

Some of the important nutrients missing in refined grains are iron, thiamine, riboflavin, and niacin. The Enrichment Act of 1942 required that these nutrients be returned to the flour. However, the nutrients added come from a synthetic, not a natural source. Further, enrichment does not remedy all the deficits created by refining grain. Research has shown that other nutrients are lost, including fiber, trace minerals, magnesium, zinc, folic acid, vitamin B_6, and essential fatty acids.

Refined flour products present a threat for everyone, but especially for diabetics, because they convert very rapidly to glucose since there is no fiber to slow down the absorption rate. Blood-sugar levels can rise very rapidly.

Grains should be eaten in their whole, complex form and the best breads are the seven-grain, sprouted, flourless breads. These breads are not made from flour. Grains are sprouted, dried, and made into loaves, thereby retaining all the complex nutrients inherent in whole grains. These delicious breads are packed with nutrients and fiber. Their sugars are released very slowly into the bloodstream, avoiding the danger in diabetics of rapid blood-sugar elevation. Sprouted-grain breads are also more alkaline than other breads, a metabolic benefit. People with allergies to grains can often eat these breads, because the sprouting process consumes gluten and other grain subfractions that cause most allergic reactions.

Read the label on every package of food you buy. Avoid those foods containing enriched flour, refined wheat flour, bleached flour, unbleached pastry flour, and high-gluten flour. These foods contain simple carbohydrates, which are rapidly absorbed and will raise blood-sugar levels.

Another ingredient to avoid is any oil added to packaged foods. This may include canola, soy, sunflower, safflower, cottonseed, corn, coconut, and palm oil. (Organic, non-hydrogenated coconut oil is fine to use, but it will not be the type you find in most processed food.) These oils will have been processed, refined, and heated during the manufacture of the food, all of which damage the oils and form dangerous trans-fatty acids. These oxidized fats damage the walls of arteries and interfere with the action of insulin. Foods prepared with olive oil or butter are better choices, because these fats resist heating and are not degraded.

Avoid also chemicals, preservatives, colorings, and of course, sugars. High-fructose corn syrup has a high glucose content and will rapidly elevate the blood sugar.

Breakfast Suggestions and Combinations

One

Hot rolled oats (long-cooking) or steel-cut oats with xylitol or stevia and soy or almond milk

Fresh fruit and Ezekiel (a sprouted grain bread) toast with butter

Two

Eggs (fertile, cage-free) scrambled or poached (Poached or soft boiled is best.)

Ezekiel toast, or 100% whole-wheat toast with butter

Fresh fruit

Three

French toast with xylitol maple syrup, fruit syrup, or jam (see recipes)

Organic, plain, non-fat yogurt or cottage cheese with fruit

Four

Hot steel-cut oats with xylitol or stevia and soy or almond milk

Ezekiel toast with butter

Fresh fruit

Five

Fruit salad (see recipes)
Ezekiel toast with butter

Six

Omelet with goat cheese
Fresh fruit
Almond orange muffin (see recipes)

Seven

Yogurt with granola (see recipes)
Fresh fruit
Hot chocolate (see recipes)

Eight

Poached apples with nuts and flaxseeds (see recipes)
Ezekiel toast with butter

Nine

Cottage cheese pancakes (see recipe)
Fresh fruit

Yogurt Cheese

(Replacement for cream cheese)

32 oz. of organic, plain, non-fat yogurt
Line a large strainer with cheesecloth.

Place yogurt in strainer and place strainer over a pot, allowing liquid to drain into pot. Cover with a saucer and place in refrigerator for 8–24 hrs, until yogurt is consistency of cheese.

YIELDS 2 cups cheese substitute for cream cheese, butter, mayo, or sour cream

DID YOU KNOW?

Soy protein is a *complete protein,* having as many amino acids as a steak, and is therefore a good animal protein substitute! Also, it is alkaline, not acid—thereby reducing the acid load on the kidneys.

Granola

½ *cup oat flakes, non-instant*
½ *cup rye flakes, non-instant*
2 *Tbsp. brown-rice syrup*
1 *Tbsp. water*

2 *Tbsp. whole sesame seeds*
2 *Tbsp. chopped almonds*
1 *Tbsp. ghee* or coconut oil*

Preheat oven to 350 degrees. Place oats and rye flakes on a dry cookie sheet. Bake 10–15 minutes. Mix brown-rice syrup and water and toss with nuts, seeds, and oat and rye flakes. Place a thin film of coconut oil on a cookie sheet and spread granola mixture evenly over pan. Bake for 20 minutes, stirring every 5 minutes. When finished cooking, stir ghee or coconut oil evenly through granola. Serve with chopped apple, raspberries, or blueberries and soy or almond milk. Can also be sprinkled over non-fat organic yogurt.

*Ghee is clarified butter and has been used in India for hundreds of years. It is much healthier than cooking with vegetable oils. (Olive oil is okay.)

DID YOU KNOW?

MCTs (Medium chain triglycerides) found in coconut oil are different from other fats. They are burned as a quick source of energy and are therefore not generally stored in body tissue. Studies have shown coconut oil to have little effect on cholesterol levels. Commercial coconut oil is not recommended as it is usually bleached and hydrogenated. Healthy, organic coconut oil may be purchased from a number of companies (see resource section).

French Toast

2 eggs (fertile, cage-free, omega-rich)
2 Tbsp. soy or almond milk
½ tsp. vanilla (can use natural
  maple, orange, or lemon flavor)

½ tsp. cinnamon
2 slices 7-grain sprouted bread

Mix eggs, milk, vanilla, and cinnamon (use wire whisk). Dip bread into egg batter and cook on medium-hot skillet that has a thin film of olive or coconut oil on it. Brown both sides and serve with xylitol maple syrup.

SERVES 2

Fruit Syrup

1 pkg. unsweetened frozen berries
(Or a low-glycemic fruit of choice)

Thaw berries, place in pan, and cover with water (approx. 1 in. above fruit). Add xylitol or stevia to taste. Bring to a low simmer.
  In a bowl, combine:

1–2 Tbsp. kudzu (as you would cornstarch)
1–2 Tbsp. water

Add to syrup to desired thickness and simmer 1–2 minutes.
  Serve over French toast, yogurt, or crepes.
  This syrup may be made thicker and used as a jam.

Cinnamon Toast

2 slices 7-grain sprouted bread or
100% whole-wheat bread

Combine:

1 tbsp. xylitol
½ tsp. cinnamon (or to taste)

Toast bread lightly. Butter toast with organic butter. Sprinkle with cinnamon-xylitol mixture and place under broiler for about 1 minute.

Xylitol Maple Syrup

2 cups water
¾ cup xylitol (use a bit more or less as desired)

2 tsp. natural, alcohol-free maple flavoring
Pinch of Celtic sea salt

Simmer 1–2 minutes
    In a bowl, combine:

2 Tbsp. Kudzu (as you would cornstarch)
2 Tbsp. water

Add to simmering syrup to thicken to your preference.
    Simmer 1–2 minutes more, cool, and serve.
    Use immediately.

Omelet with Veggies

2 eggs (fertile, cage-free)
2 tsp. water
¾ cup combined chopped fa-vorite veggies (at least 3 types, low glycemic)

½ tsp. onion powder
1 Tbsp. olive oil
Pinch Celtic sea salt

Sauté veggies in olive oil; set aside. Mix eggs with water and whisk lightly. Heat pan to medium heat. Place thin film of olive oil in pan and add eggs, lifting edges of omelet as it cooks. Do not overcook; leave moist. Slide from pan and add veggies. Fold in half and serve. YIELDS 1 omelet.
    Variation: Before removing omelet from pan, add 1 Tbsp. grated goat cheese and/or some avocado bits. Remove pan from stove, cover 1 minute, and allow cheese to melt. Remove omelet from pan, add veggies, and fold over.

Breakfast Yogurt Salad

Cut into small pieces:
1 organic apple
1 organic pear
½ cup organic fresh or frozen
  blueberries or strawberries
2 Tbsp. each: raw sunflower and
  pumpkin seeds, lightly toasted
sesame seeds, and almonds.
(These may be ground up for small children.)

4–6 Tbsp. of organic plain non-
fat yogurt

Mix fruit, seeds, and nuts. Stir in yogurt and enjoy.

SERVES 2–4

DID YOU KNOW?

Yogurt has friendly bacteria, which keep unhealthy bacteria (such as yeast and candida albicans) from growing out of control in the intestine and colon. Yogurt also promotes the production of many important B vitamins. Only natural organic yogurt will contain such friendly bacteria. You can purchase it at your local health food store.

Hot Chocolate

1 cup warm soy or almond milk
Add 1–2 tsp. xylitol chocolate sauce to taste

Orange Almond Muffin

2 cups ground almonds
½ cup whole-wheat flour
½ tsp. baking soda
1 tsp. cinnamon
⅛ tsp. Celtic sea salt

¼ cup unsweetened applesauce
1 Tbsp. orange zest (grated orange peel)
½ cup brown-rice syrup
2 eggs

Grind nuts in a coffee grinder. Place them in a bowl with flour, soda, cinnamon, and salt. Blend together well. Add eggs and syrup and mix well. Add applesauce (more or less, until proper muffin consistency). Place paper liners in muffin tins. Fill half full with batter and bake at 350 degrees for approximately 25 minutes.

YIELDS 8–10 muffins

Poached Apples with Flaxseeds and Nuts

2 apples, chopped

Poach in ¼ cup water with ½ tsp. cinnamon (or to taste) Add: 2 tsp. xylitol and cook only until tender but still firm. Cool!

Stir in ¼ cup chopped walnuts or other nuts and 1 Tbsp. freshly ground flaxseed (you can use a small coffee grinder). Mix well and place in serving bowls.

SERVES 2

Serve with Gourmet Cream Sauce.

Cottage Cheese Pancakes

3 eggs	*1 Tbsp. coconut oil or melted butter*
1 cup low-fat cottage cheese	*2 Tbsp. 100% whole-wheat flour*

Beat eggs. Add to cottage cheese and mix together. Add oil and flour. Mix.
Heat griddle with a little coconut oil until quite hot. Place ¼ cup batter on hot griddle and spread it out a bit.
Cook 1–1½ minutes on each side.
Serve with unsweetened applesauce (a little cinnamon sprinkled on top is good) or use unsweetened Apple Butter or homemade xylitol fruit syrup or jam.

MAKES 6–8 pancakes

Lunches for School or at Home

Sandwiches:

Use whole-wheat pita bread, 100% whole-wheat bread, or Ezekiel bread.

Add chicken, turkey, roast beef, or peanut, almond, macadamia, or cashew butter, or tahini (organic). Use homemade xylitol jam or rice syrup.

Goat cheeses with lettuce and avocado.

Scrambled eggs or tuna.

Mustard, homemade egg-free mayonnaise, or yogurt may be used in sandwiches.

Egg-Free Mayonnaise

¾ cups soft tofu	*½ tsp. tamari soy sauce*
2 Tbsp. brown-rice vinegar (sugar-free)	*1 Tbsp. virgin olive oil*
1 tsp. Dijon mustard	

Combine first 4 ingredients in blender on low speed until creamy. At a higher speed, begin adding the olive oil and blend until thoroughly combined.

One

Hard-boiled eggs. (fertile, cage-free)
Celery sticks with peanut butter or almond butter or yogurt
cheese (see recipes)
Orange of apple sections
Almond milk

Two

Soy beans in pods. (Edamame; see frozen section in grocery
or health food store)
Fruit cups with finger-sized pieces of different fruits
Raw nuts or oil-free soy nuts
Cucumber pieces and cherry tomatoes

Three

Turkey salad in whole-wheat pita pocket with lettuce and
tomato
Soy milk
Apple wedges

Four

Grilled goat cheese sandwich on Ezekiel bread
Pickles (unsweetened)
Cherry tomatoes
Soy milk

Five

Boca Burger on toasted Ezekiel bread or sprouted buns with
lettuce, tomato
BBQ Beans
Iced tea with stevia (see beverages)

Six

Roast beef sandwich on Ezekiel with mustard
Oil-free soy nuts
Soy milk
Strawberries

Seven

BBQ Bean sandwiches in whole-wheat pita pocket (pack beans
separately if taking to school)
Slices of goat cheese
Cherry tomato
Soy milk

Eight

Bean and pasta soup
Rye Vita crackers
Goat cheese cubes
Apple wedges

Nine

Egg salad sandwich (made with homemade mayo on pita
bread)
Celery and pickle sticks
Soy milk

Ten

Individual pizzas on sprouted bagels (see recipe)
Small green salad
Iced tea

Eleven

Almond butter with brown-rice syrup sandwich on toasted
Ezekiel
Soy milk
Orange sections

Twelve

Tuna sandwich with homemade egg-free mayo on Ezekiel or
pita bread
Celery sticks
Cherry tomatoes
Iced tea

Beverages

Fruity iced teas, sweetened with stevia or xylitol. This can be frozen in a plastic spring water bottle (fill ¾ full) and put in lunch in place of ice pack.

Almond or soy milks, chocolate, carob, or vanilla (available in small sizes)

Homemade lemonade, sweetened with stevia or xylitol

Dinner Recipes

Chicken Moutarde with couscous, steamed veggies, green salad, water or herbal teas

Omelets with veggies and a salad

Lasagna with ground beef (organic) with veggies and a green salad

Tofu veggie stir-fry with green salad

Boca Burgers with lettuce and tomato, baked BBQ beans, and green salad

Herbal chicken patties with mock mashed potatoes and green salad

Pizza with green salad

Chicken soup and green salad with Ezekiel garlic toast

Tuna casserole, sliced tomato, and green salad

Bean and pasta soup with green salad and sprouted rolls

Baked fish with couscous and steamed veggies

Chili with ground turkey breast and green salad

Spaghetti with ground beef, green salad, and garlic toast

Lemon turkey patties, steamed veggies with goat cheese, green salad

Spaghetti with shrimp, salad, and steamed veggies

DID YOU KNOW?

80% of Americans do not eat the necessary amount of fruits and vegetables required for good health!

Bean Pasta Soup

1 16-ounce can butter beans, drained, or freshly made	1 cup celery, chopped
7 cups non-fat chicken broth	2 tsp. olive oil
1/4 cup whole-wheat macaroni	1/4 cup water
1 large sweet potato, chopped	1 bay leaf
1 large onion, chopped	1 tsp. marjoram
1 zucchini, chopped	1 Tbsp. parsley
1 tsp. each onion and garlic powder	1/2 cup tofu (blend with 1 cup of broth)

Sauté celery and onion for 5 minutes. Add 1/4 cup water. Add sweet potato, zucchini, bay leaf, and garlic/onion powder. Simmer covered for 10 minutes. Add all of this to chicken broth with canned beans and macaroni. Add marjoram and parsley and tofu mixture. Simmer 6–7 minutes until pasta is done, yet still firm (al dente).

SERVES 8

Chicken Soup

2 cans undiluted chicken broth	1 tsp. thyme
1 medium sweet potato, cut up	1 tsp. basil
2 stalks celery, sliced	1/2 tsp. garlic or onion powder
1 onion, chopped small	1 cup cooked chicken pieces
1 bay leaf (remove when finished cooking)	1 cup cooked barley

Simmer 15–20 minutes.

SERVES 4

Lasagna

Sauté in 1 Tbsp. olive oil until cooked (but still crisp):

1 crushed garlic clove   *1 cup chopped favorite veggies*
½ cup chopped onion

Add:

1 lb. ground turkey breast   *1 tsp. Celtic sea salt*

Cook until done.
    Add:

1 pound can of tomatoes (or 6 fresh)   *2 tsp. xylitol*
8 oz. can of Muir Glen tomato sauce   *½ cup unsweetened applesauce*

Cook until well blended.
    Cook: 8 oz. of whole-grain lasagna noodles
    Stir together: 4 oz. of yogurt cheese, 1 cup cottage cheese
    Lightly oil 13" x 9" pan with olive oil. Place a layer of noodles, then meat sauce, and then cheese. Repeat each ingredient a second time.
    Bake at 350 degrees for 45 minutes.
    Add ½ cup grated goat cheese on top the last 10 minutes.

SERVES 8

Chicken Moutarde

6 single chicken breasts, washed and dried (skins removed)

Place in baking dish and pour juice of one lemon over chicken.

Blend together in a bowl:

½ cup brown-rice syrup   *½ cup Dijon mustard*

Drizzle over chicken.
Bake at 350 degrees 50 minutes to 1 hour.
Baste every 15 minutes with the sauce in the pan.

SERVES 6

Herbal Chicken Patties

Place: 3 Tbsp. fat-free chicken broth in a large frying pan. Bring to simmer.
Sprinkle chicken patties (to taste) with:

Parsley   *Ground sage is also very good if desired.*
Onion and garlic powder

Add to pan and simmer 2 minutes or cook each side until done.

Lemon Turkey Patties

Put juice of ½ large lemon in non-stick frying pan. Add 2 turkey patties to medium-hot pan. Sprinkle with onion and garlic powder. Simmer 2 minutes on each side. Lemon juice will be completely absorbed.

SERVES 2

Broiled Fish

2 lbs. sole or other fish fillets	*3 Tbsp. chopped green onion*
2 Tbsp. lemon juice	*¼ tsp. Celtic sea salt*
½ cup Parmesan cheese	*¼–½ tsp. cayenne pepper (to*
2–3 Tbsp. melted butter	*taste)*
3 Tbsp. homemade mayonnaise	
(made with olive oil)	

Pat fillets with paper towel. Place them in an oiled baking pan. Sprinkle or brush with lemon juice. Let stand 10–15 minutes. Combine remaining ingredients. Set aside. Broil fish 4 inches from heat for 6–8 minutes until fish flakes easily. Remove from oven and spread the cheese mixture evenly over fish. Broil another 2–3 minutes until lightly brown.

SERVES 4–6

DID YOU KNOW?

Encouraging children to eat fish at an earlier age will help to guarantee greater amounts of certain "essential fats" that children are very often deficient in. These fats are essential for new cell development.

Tuna and Veggie Casserole

Cook 1 pkg. whole-wheat macaroni or buckwheat spirals. Set aside. In frying pan, sauté 1 chopped medium onion in 1 Tbsp. olive oil.
Add:

1 can of salt-free chicken broth and simmer 5 minutes.

Rub sides and bottom of casserole dish with olive oil. Fill with cooked noodles.
Add:

2 cans water-packed tuna, drained
½ pkg. each of organic frozen peas, corn, and lima beans

Sprinkle with garlic and onion powder to taste. Whip 3 eggs with 3 Tbsp. soy milk and pour over mixture. Add soup and onions and stir to blend all ingredients well. Cover top with ½ cup grated goat cheese. Bake at 350 degrees for 45 minutes.

SERVES 6

Chili

3 Tbsp. olive oil	*2 Tbsp. tomato paste*
1 large onion, chopped	*1 cup fresh or frozen corn*
1 clove garlic, crushed	*4 cups dried, cooked kidney or pinto beans*
1 green pepper (optional), diced	*½ tsp. chili powder (or to taste)*
1 lb. ground turkey breast	*¼ tsp. cumin powder*
2 cups non-fat chicken broth	*1 tsp. Celtic sea salt*

Sauté onion, garlic, and green pepper until soft. Add 1 lb. ground turkey breast and cook until done. Add broth, tomato paste, and corn. Mash 2 cups of beans and add to pot with other beans and seasonings. Simmer 30–40 minutes.

SERVES 6

Pasta Sauce

Sauté in olive oil:
1 onion chopped, until done. Add 1 cup sliced mushrooms and cook 3–5 minutes. Add ¼ pound lean ground beef per person, cook until done (to your preference). Add this meat mixture to a jar of your favorite pasta sauce (sugar- and oil-free; olive oil is okay). Serve over whole-grain pasta cooked al dente. Sprinkle with non-fat Parmesan cheese.

SERVES 4–6

DID YOU KNOW?

Tomato sauce is one of the best sources of lycopene—a powerful antioxidant that makes the tomato red. Lycopene offers great protection for the eyes and vision.

Pizza

Cut sprouted bagel in half. Spread with tomato sauce and sprinkle on grated goat cheese. Add some chopped, fresh basil and place under broiler until cheese bubbles. Optional: A little garlic or onion powder may be sprinkled on top of cheese before broiling.
Options: cooked veggies, ground chicken, turkey, or low-fat beef.

Sweet Potato Pie

Steam or bake 6 sweet potatoes. Chop 3 or 4 apples and poach in 3–4 Tbsp. water until tender. Mash sweet potatoes and spread into a 13" Pyrex baking dish.
    In a saucepan combine:

¼ cup butter
⅛ tsp. white stevia power (optional)
Poached apples
1 to 1½ cups chopped walnuts or pecans

¼ cup brown-rice syrup
¼–½ tsp. cinnamon
¼ tsp. nutmeg
Juice of 1 small lemon

Heat over low heat until butter melts. Pour mixture over sweet potatoes. Bake at 350 degrees for 30 minutes.

DID YOU KNOW?

There is a difference between sweet potatoes (acceptable for diabetics) and yams (unacceptable). Sweet potatoes have skins that are yellowish-orange whereas yams are a dark red or burgundy color.

Barbecued Beans

3 cups cooked (dried, not canned)
  beans of choice
½ chopped onion
1 grated apple
1 grated zucchini
2 Tbsp. olive oil

1 tsp. dry mustard powder
½ cup homemade BBQ sauce (see recipe)
¾ cup vegetable broth made from Dr. Jensen's Vegetable Seasoning Powder (1 tsp. in ¾ cup water)

Sauté onion in oil 3 minutes. Add apples and zucchini. Cook covered for 5 minutes. Mix with remaining ingredients. Bake covered for 45 minutes.

SERVES 6

DIGESTIBLE BEANS

Beans are notoriously difficult to digest and can cause excessive gas and bloating. By following this method of preparation the problem is usually eliminated:

Soak beans overnight. In the morning pour off water and rinse the beans. Add new water and heat beans at a low simmer for 10 to 15 minutes. Then pour the water off. Add new water again. Add seasoning and continue cooking the beans until done. This should minimize the digestive problems that beans can cause.

The difficulty with beans results from enzyme inhibitors that are present in the hard outer shell of the bean. Nature wisely equipped the beans with a certain chemical that prevents the spoilage that would normally occur when whole foods are stored. Fresh whole foods eventually spoil, mold, rot, and go back into nature. This breakdown process results from the enzymes present in fresh food. The enzyme inhibitors in beans preserve the beans by blocking enzymatic activity. However, when we eat beans, these same inhibitors interfere with our own digestive enzymes. Uncomfortable gas and bloating result.

BBQ Sauce

⅔ cup tomato sauce
2 cloves crushed garlic
1 Tbsp. brown-rice syrup
2 Tbsp. lemon juice
2 Tbsp. finely chopped onions

1 tsp. basil
½ tsp. chili power (or to taste)
¼ tsp. cumin powder
⅛ tsp. ginger powder

In a frying pan sauté garlic and onions in a small amount of olive oil until soft. Add the remaining ingredients and simmer for 3–4 minutes.

Mock Mashed Potatoes

1 large head of cauliflower cut into pieces   *Celtic sea salt to taste*
¼ cup organic plain non-fat yogurt   *Chopped green onion or parsley for garnish*

Cook cauliflower until tender, drain, and puree in a blender. Add yogurt and salt and blend thoroughly. Reheat and serve garnished with onion and parsley.
    Variation: Place in baking dish and sprinkle with grated goat cheese. Place under broiler for 1–2 minutes until cheese melts.

SERVES 4

DID YOU KNOW?

Cruciferous vegetables (i.e., broccoli, cabbage, cauliflower, brussel sprouts) are high in certain phytochemicals that protect us from different forms of cancer.

Dessert Recipes

Nutty Oatmeal Cookies

½ cup soft butter   *½ cup ground almonds*
⅔ cup xylitol   *½ tsp. baking soda*
1 egg, beaten   *½ tsp. Celtic sea salt*
½ cup organic peanut butter   *1 cup rolled oats*
1½ tsp. vanilla   *½ cup chopped dry-roasted*
½ cup whole-wheat flour   *peanuts or fresh walnuts*

Cream butter and add xylitol. Add egg; beat well. Stir in peanut butter and vanilla; beat until smooth. Combine flour, almond meal, soda, and salt; mix well and add slowly to butter/xylitol mixture. Add oats and nuts; blend. Drop by teaspoons onto greased cookie sheet. Flatten slightly with fork. Bake at 350 degrees for 12–14 minutes.

YIELDS 3 dozen

Apple Crisp

2 cups peeled apples, sliced
2 tsp. cinnamon
Pinch of nutmeg
½ cup oatmeal
2 tsp. virgin olive oil or
   coconut oil

2 Tbsp. melted butter
¼ cup water
¼ cup ground almonds
¼–½ cup walnuts (chopped)
2–4 Tbsp. xylitol (depending on sweetness of apples)

Layer apples in an 8-inch-square baking dish. Pour water over fruit and combine ground almonds, oatmeal, walnuts, and oil. Combine cinnamon, nutmeg, and xylitol. Sprinkle over apples. Cover apples with the oatmeal mixture. Drizzle on melted butter. Bake at 350 degrees for 30–40 minutes or until brown.

SERVES 4

Poached Fruit

A good way to use overripe fruit is to combine any of your low-glycemic fruits. Chop and place in a pan. Add about one inch of water (do not use too much). Add 1 Tbsp. of xylitol (or to taste) and ¼ tsp. cinnamon (optional). Simmer 5–6 minutes. This fruit is delicious with yogurt, French toast, or cream sauce, or chopped toasted almonds.

Frozen Yogurt

2 cups plain yogurt	*1–2 Tbsp. xylitol or brown-rice*
1 quart frozen berries, peaches,	*syrup or stevia (to taste)*
cherries, or any low-glycemic fruit	

Place one cup of yogurt in a blender. Gradually add fruit and remaining yogurt, alternating them. Add sweetener and blend until thickened. Pour into a container and place in the freezer until ready to eat. This ice cream should be eaten soon after making. Do not refreeze.

SERVES 4

Great with xylitol chocolate sauce and chopped toasted almonds!

Jiffy Cake

¾ cup xylitol	*1½ cups whole-wheat flour*
¼ cup cocoa powder	*½ tsp. Celtic sea salt*
1 tsp. soda	

Sift all of these together into an ungreased 8-inch-square baking pan.

Add:

1 Tbsp. apple-cider vinegar	*⅓ cup melted butter*
1 Tbsp. vanilla	*1 cup cold water*

Stir until no lumps remain. Bake at 350 degrees for 30–35 minutes until a knife comes out clean.

This cake makes a quick and tasty dessert or treat. Lovely with whipped cream or homemade raspberry syrup.

Brownies

½ *cup whole-wheat flour*
½ *cup almonds, ground fine*
½ *tsp. baking powder*
¾ *tsp. salt*
2 *eggs*
½ *tsp. while stevia powder*

2 *squares (1 oz. each) unsweetened*
   chocolate, melted and cooled
1 *tsp. vanilla*
½ *cup chopped nuts*
⅓ *cup melted butter*
½ *cup brown-rice syrup*

Heat oven to 350 degrees. Sift flour and ground almonds with baking powder and salt. Beat eggs and add stevia. Stir in ground almonds. Add melted butter, chocolate, vanilla, and brown-rice syrup. Mix and stir in flour mixture. Add nuts. Oil an 8-inch baking pan with butter. Pour in batter and spread evenly. Bake 20–25 minutes (do not overcook). Test with a clean knife. Cool on cake rack for 5 minutes. Cut into squares.

MAKES 16 brownies

Peach Tart

1¾ *cups whole-wheat flour*
2 *Tbsp. xylitol*
½ *tsp. salt*
¼ *tsp. baking powder*

½ *cup butter*
4–6 *sliced peaches (fresh or*
   frozen, or canned packed in water)

Combine together:

½–⅔ *cup xylitol*
1–1½ *tsp. cinnamon*

2 *egg yolks*
1 *cup soy milk*

In a bowl blend together:
   Flour and salt, 2 Tbsp. xylitol, and baking powder.
   Cut in butter until flour looks like pebbles. Press mixture evenly into bottom of an 8-inch-square baking dish. Arrange sliced peaches on top of crust. Sprinkle with xylitol–cinnamon mixture. Bake at 400 degrees for 15 minutes. Mix egg yolks and soy milk. Pour over peaches. Bake 30 minutes or longer.

Lemon Pudding

½ cup xylitol
¼ tsp. white stevia powder
¼ cup kudzu
1½ cups cold water

3 egg yolks
¼ cup fresh lemon juice
zest from 1 large lemon
1 Tbsp. butter

In bowl, beat egg yolks well; set aside. Place water, xylitol, stevia, and kudzu in a pan. Blend well with wire whisk. Simmer until thickened, stirring constantly while cooking, as kudzu can become lumpy. Slowly add 4 Tbsp. of hot liquid to beaten egg yolks (1 Tbsp. at a time). Then add this mixture to the liquid in the pan, again using the wire whisk to mix well. Add lemon juice and butter, blending well. Pour into 6 small pudding cups and cool.

SERVES 6
May also be used for lemon meringue pie.

Almond Cookies

2 Tbsp. soft butter
¾ cup xylitol
¾ cup almond butter
2 egg whites
1 Tbsp. vanilla

1½ cups whole-wheat flour
½ cup chopped, toasted almonds
½ tsp. baking soda
¼ Tbsp. sea salt

Heat oven to 370 degrees. Oil cookie sheet with butter or coconut oil. Combine butter and half the xylitol and beat until creamy. Add the remainder of the xylitol, almond butter, egg whites, and vanilla. Beat until mixed. Blend flour, soda, and salt. Combine with wet mixture. Add almonds and blend. Spoon rounded tsps. onto cookie sheet 2 inches apart. Flatten each with a fork (criss-cross). Do not flatten too much! Bake at 375 degrees for 7–10 minutes. Cool.

MAKES 4 dozen

Yogurt Dessert

1 cup non-fat, plain organic yogurt
1/4–1/2 tsp. almond, vanilla, or
    orange extract
1–2 tsp. xylitol (or 2–3 drops stevia)
    to taste

1 Tbsp. chopped, toasted
    almonds and/or toasted sesame
    seeds

Mix yogurt, extract, and sweetener. Top with almonds and/or sesame seeds.

SERVES 2

Variation: brown-rice syrup may be substituted for xylitol or stevia.

Gourmet Cream Sauce

1 pint organic, low-fat cottage cheese
1 tsp. almond or vanilla extract
(to taste)

1–2 tsp. soy or almond milk
2–3 drops stevia or 1–2 Tbsp.
    xylitol (to taste)

Place all ingredients in blender. Blend until smooth. Keep refrigerated. Serve over fruit, crepes, fruit salads, French toast, or poached fruit.

For variations: Omit sweeteners and extracts and add curry powder or soy sauce to taste. Serve over veggies with toasted sesame seeds. Also good over fish or couscous. Use orange or lemon extract instead of vanilla or almond. Also good with cinnamon added.

Fruity Gelatin

3 cups sweetened* fruit-flavored tea   *2 Tbsp. agar-agar flakes*

Simmer 2 minutes and cool.
Place 4 cups low-glycemic fruit in bottom of 8-inch-square glass pan. Pour tea mixture over fruit. Sprinkle chopped nuts of choice over top. Refrigerate for 2–3 hours.

YIELDS approx. 10 servings

* with stevia or xylitol

Xylitol Chocolate Sauce

1 cup water
½ cup xylitol
¼ cup organic, fat-free powdered milk

½ cup low-fat, caffeine-free cocoa powder
2–3 Tbsp. melted butter
1 tsp. vanilla extract

Place all ingredients in a pan and blend well with a wire whisk. Place over medium heat and bring to a boil. Reduce heat and simmer on low for 4–5 minutes. Cool and store in refrigerator. Serve over homemade frozen yogurt, fruit, plain yogurt, or dessert crepes. Also may be added to soy, goat, or almond milk to make a cold or hot chocolate drink.

Crepes

3 whole eggs
2 Tbsp. whole-wheat flour

1–2 Tbsp. soy, rice, or skim milk
1–2 Tbsp. water

Beat eggs with flour until smooth. Add milk and water, starting with one tablespoon of each and adding more as needed. The batter will be quite thin. Heat a small non-stick sauté pan over medium heat. Pour ¼ cup of batter into pan and swirl around until bottom is coated. Cook for 2–3 minutes until lightly browned.

Remove from pan and fill with 2 or 3 tablespoons of poached fruit and top with cream sauce.

MAKES 4 crepes

Variations: May be filled with yogurt cheese and topped with xylitol fruit syrup or jam. Or fill with sautéed veggies and top with the curried cream sauce.

Nut Butter Balls

1 cup organic peanut, almond, or cashew butter, or tahini	*¼ cup protein powder* *2–3 Tbsp. brown-rice syrup*

Blend together in a bowl and form into bite-sized balls. Children also enjoy helping to make these treats—a nice family project.

DID YOU KNOW?

Research has proven that only 1% of children between the ages of 2 and 19 eat a diet adequate to meet the recommended daily requirements of nutrients. Soda pop can leach calcium and magnesium out of children's growing bones, weakening them. These drinks also expose children to the aluminum heavy metal, which is leached into these acid drinks from the cans they come in.

Snacks

1. Raw sunflower and pumpkin seeds (purchased in sealed bags and kept in freezer).
2. Raw almonds (and other raw nuts, including oil-free soy nuts; keep in freezer).
3. Celery with peanut butter, almond butter, or yogurt cheese.
4. Protein drink (see recipe) or Revival Soy Drink, Naturade Soy Protein, Now Soy Protein, or Nutribiotic Rice Protein.

5. Apples with raw almond butter or goat cheese.
6. Hummus dip (without oil except for olive oil, which is okay) with vegetables or crackers.
7. Wasa crackers with raw almond butter, peanut butter, or goat cheese (keep refrigerated).
8. Ryvita crackers with avocado and goat cheese.
9. Two or three pieces of fruit per day, perferably organic. Avoid high-glycemic-index fruits like bananas, watermelons, and grapes.
10. Half a sandwich: chicken, avodaco, raw almond butter or other nut butters with brown-rice syrup, scrambled egg, or grilled goat cheese. Use sprouted breads and mustard, plain non-fat yogurt, or homemade mayo (see recipe).
11. Soy-protein wafers.
12. One slice sprouted, flourless toast with brown-rice syrup, nut butter or tahini, or xylitol jam.
13. Iced teas sweetened with stevia or xylitol (in place of soda and juice). Comes in sports bottle for outings.
14. Non-fat, organic cottage cheese or plain white yogurt with low-glycemic fruit.
15. Raw soybeans in the pod (freezer section) (also known as Edamame). Remove from pod after cooking if easier for the child.
16. Plain, organic yogurt (non-fat) with brown-rice syrup and chopped nuts.
17. Hard-boiled eggs.
18. Popsicles made from teas (see 13 above).
19. Whole-wheat pretzels (no oil).
20. Homemade cookies (see recipes).
21. Xylitol gum and mints.
22. Cinnamon toast (see recipe).
23. Sugatrol RX™ (see Resource Section).

These snacks can easily be carried on outings, to movies, and to sports events.

Yogurt Dill Dip

1 cup organic, non-fat yogurt   *1–2 tsp. fresh or dried dill*
½ tsp. onion powder (to taste)

Serve with raw veggies or over fish.
Great for after-school snacks or parties.

Drinks

Protein Drink

2 cups almond milk   *2 tsp. vanilla*
¾ cup ice chips   *1 tsp. cardamom powder*
2 tsp. brown-rice syrup   *¼ tsp. nutmeg*
Stevia or xylitol to taste   *½ tsp. cinnamon*
4 Tbsp. unsweetened protein powder   *2 Tbsp. flaxseed, freshly ground*

Blend until frothy.

SERVES 2

Protein Drink

½ cup water   *2 Tbsp. unsweetened protein powder*
½ cup plain yogurt   *Xylitol or stevia to taste*
½ cup frozen berries or cherries

Almond Milk

¼ cup almonds   *⅛ tsp. Celtic sea salt*
2 cups warm, pure water

Soak nuts overnight. Drain and throw soak water away. Remove skins of nuts if desired. Blend nuts with 2 cups warm water and sea salt. Use as is or strain. Store in refrigerator.

Appendix I

PROPER EATING/SHOPPING GUIDE

Foods	Products to Look For at Your Local Health Food Store
Applesauce Unsprayed, unsweet-ened, organic	*Solana Gold* and many other good organic brands
Beans	Eden, Westbrae Natural, American Prairie
Breads Sprouted, flourless are best	*Food for Life:* Ezekiel, flourless, sprouted *Oasis:* flourless, sprouted English muffins, 5-grain, sprouted 100% whole wheat or whole rye; no white flour
Butters, Nut Unsprayed only	*Arrowhead Mills:* raw, organic is the best (see Resource Section)
Cereal/Grains Organic: whole & un-sprayed	*Arrowhead Mills, Bob's Red Mill, Old Wessex:* Quinoa, oat groats, steel-cut oats, old-fashioned oatmeal, wheat berries, Barley, buckwheat, brown rice* (corn meal/millet not recommended for diabetics) *see glycemic index
Cheese Organic preferred Avoid for children under 2.	*Alta Dena* or *Horizon:* organic cottage cheese, organic mozzarella, goat cheese, feta cheese, and Parmesan cheese

Foods	Products to Look For At Your Local Health Food Store
Cocoa Powder Organic preferred	*Wonderslim*
Crackers	Kauli, Finn Crisp, Ryvita, Wasa
Dairy Products Cow's milk not recommended for children under 2 years of age. If you give milk to older children, a non-homogenized (cream at the top) milk is a superior product. It can be found in some health food stores. Skim milk is also acceptable. Goat milk can be used for children of any age. For formula, goat milk must be diluted ⅔ milk to ⅓ water. Vitamin and mineral supplementation is necessary. Soy milk is acceptable for children over 2.	Alta Dena and Horizon produce good organic milk products. The only non-homogenized milk products that we know of are Claravale Farms and Brown Cow yogurt. Meyenberg goat milk is available in health food stores and supermarkets. Goat milk is naturally homogenized.
Eggs Fertile/cage free	Many brands. *Gold Circle Farms* for DHA eggs. See "The Truth About Eggs" page 99.
Fish Canned, organic	See Resource Section
Flour Whole Grain (refrigerate/freeze)	*Arrowhead Mills* (unsprayed) purchased in sealed bags. Kept in refrigerator or freezer.
Healthy Candies	Sugatrol RX™ Bar See Resource Section
Ice Cream	See recipe under Desserts.

Foods	Products to Look For At Your Local Health Food Store
Mayonnaise	Made with virgin olive oil See recipe under Lunches.
Meats Organic only	Chemical/hormone-free chicken and tur-key, red meat. Tempeh and tofu are good substitutes for meat. Call your local health food store. *Shelton Farms Chicken and Turkey, Diestel Turkey.* Available in health food stores and some supermarkets. as well as mail order (see Resource Section)
Milk Substitutes Plain, without sweeteners	*Eden Soy:* soy milk (not recom-mended for children under 2 years). *West Soy:* soy milk (best for children if fortified with calcium & magnesium (not recommended for children under 2 years). *Almond Milk:* see recipe, or Pacific brand.
Nuts & Seeds Raw, unsalted, and in sealed bags. Keep in freezer to protect oils.	Several brands. Do not purchase from bins in the market.
Oils Unrefined: no heating, filtering, or bleaching. Organic in dark, light-proof bottles. Flaxseed oil must be kept re-frigerated.	Tree of Life Oils and *Omega Nutrition:* olive, flaxseed oil, sesame, coconut, and saf-flower (the highest quality oils obtainable). Call Omega Nutrition: 1-800-661-3529 Extra virgin olive oil. Many brands (see Resource Section)
Pancake & Bake Mixes No oil	Buckwheat mixes and 100% whole-grain mixes

Foods	Products to Look For At Your Local Health Food Store
Pasta	*DeBole's, Rummo, Westbrae, Papadini,* and *Eden.* Buckwheat, 100% whole wheat, Jerusalem artichoke are recommended. *Power Protein Pasta* from Crum Creek Mills, 1-888-607-3500
Protein Powders	*Nutribiotic Rice Powder, Revival, Naturade,* and *Now* soy protein
Soft Drinks Avoid these as they deplete calcium and magnesium levels.	Instead use: iced herbal and green teas and sweeten with stevia or xylitol. Filtered water
Spices and Flavorings Buy non-irradiated spices. Use fresh herbs when available.	*Spice Hunter* *Dr. Jensen's:* broth and seasonings *Bragg's:* amino acids Garlic and onion powder, unsalted
Sugars No processed cane sugars	Instead use: brown-rice or barley syrup, or stevia (from health food stores), or xylitol (order from E.A. Labs, *www.ealabs.com*)
Sweeteners	Stevia: powder and liquid Xylitol: *Healthy Sweet* granulated; also mints and gum Brown-rice syrup from Lundberg
Thickeners	Kudzu, Agar Flakes
Tomato Products	*Muir Glen* (lined cans)
Vegetables Organic is the best	Ask for Tree of Life frozen vegetables at health food stores
Vinegars Unpasteurized cider, brown rice	*Hain, Sterling, Omega,* and other

Appendix II

RESOURCES

Companies

The following companies have a number of products listed in this resource section. Companies with only one product listed have their toll-free numbers and websites listed along with their products.

Body Wise® International
1-800-830-9596
www.bodywise.com

Carlson® Laboratories
1-800-323-4141
www.carlsonlabs.com

Carotec, Inc.
P.O. Box 9919
Naples, FL 34101
1-800-522-4279

Jarrow Formulas™
1-800-726-0886
www.jarrow.com

MegaFood
1-800-848-2542
www.megafood.com

N.E.E.D.S.
1-800-634-1380
www.needs.com

Omega Nutrition
1-800-661-3529
www.omeganutrition.com

Source Naturals®
1-800-815-2333
www.sourcenaturals.com

Tree of Life®
www.treeoflife.com

Tyler, Inc.
1-800-869-9705
www.tyler-inc.com

Important New Product Not Previously Mentioned In This Book

Protein Supplement

Proper Nutrition, Inc.
1-800-555-8868
www.propernutrition.com

Seacure®

Seacure® predigested fish protein concentrate is a whole food dietary supplement that contains all of the valuable nutrients naturally found in fish, including high quality protein, omega-3 fatty acids, vitamins, minerals, and phospholipids. Research indicates that the daily intake of fish—rich in omega-3 fatty acids— protects against impaired glucose intolerance and lowers triglyceride levels in both diabetic and non-diabetic individuals. Well-known nutritionist and author, Dr. Patrick Quillin, suggests that whole foods are always the best source of good nutrition, and he adds, "Given the fact that many people do not like the taste of fish, Seacure is the best nutrition supplement for those who cannot or will not eat fish." Dr. Quillin also says that the unique digested form of the protein in Seacure provides key peptides that have additional health benefits, particularly to the person with compromised gastrointestinal function. Proper Nutrition, Inc., the manufacturer, is also investigating numerous observations that Seacure fish protein concentrate is helpful in healing difficult diabetic ulcers. Seacure is available in 500mg capsules.

Supplements

Listed here are nutritional supplements recommended by Dr. Allan Sosin. We have endeavored to find the best companies that carry these supplements. If you cannot find a particular product at your local health food store, please contact the company directly for the names of local stores that carry it or if you need information about the product itself.

Alpha Lipoic Acid

Available from the following companies:

Carlson® Laboratories
Alpha Lipoic Acid
Available in 100mg and 300mg tablets.

Carotec
Alpha Lipoic Acid
Each capsule contains 150mg of alpha lipoic acid.

Jarrow Formulas
Alpha Lipoic Sustain 300
Each tablet contains 300 mg of alpha lipoic acid in a sustained release format to minimize gastric irritations and blood sugar fluctuations.

Source Naturals®
Alpha Lipoic Acid
For immune system support. Stimulates glutathione production. Available in 50 mg, 100 mg and 200 mg tablets.

Antioxidants

Available from the following companies:

Body Wise®
Super Cell™
Each capsule contains a wide range of antioxidants, including vitamin C, vitamin E, selenium, green tea leaf extract, L-glutathione, and more.

Carlson®
Aces®
Antioxidant Formula
Contains vitamins A, C, E and selenium in soft gels.

Aces Gold®
Contains vitamins A, C, E, selenium, and 12 more active nutrients or antioxidants, including CoQ10. Available in soft gels.

MegaFood
Antioxidant DailyFoods® Vitamin, Mineral & Herbal Formula
Contains vitamins A, C and E, zinc and selenium. DailyFoods® FoodState® nutrients are 100% Whole Food and can be taken at any time throughout the day, even on an empty stomach. Available in tablet form.

Source Naturals
Tocotrienol Antioxidant Complex™
Each softgel contains a total of 34 mg of tocotrienols (29.8 mg gamma-tocotrienol, 3 mg alpha-tocotrienol, and 1.3 mg delta-tocotrienol) and 100 IU of vitamin E (d-alpha tocopherol).

Biotin

Carlson®
Available in 1000mcg tablets

Broccoli Sprouts

Source Naturals®
Each tablet contains 120 mg broccoli sprouts standardized extract, yielding 150 mcg of sulforaphane.

Calcium

Available from the following companies:

Body Wise®
Essential Calcium+®
Calcium in tablet form, which also includes vitamin D_3, vitamin B_6, magnesium, zinc, copper, and other ingredients.

Carlson®
Chelated Cal-Mag
Two tablets contain 400mg calcium and 200mg magnesium from 333mg of calcium and magnesium chelates.

Omega Nutrition
Calcium-Magnesium Liquid (from Holistic Enterprises)
Liquid Life Essential Night Formula is a mineral-rich formula with a pleasant coconut flavor that is designed to help tissue repair and calcium assimilation while you sleep. Suitable for all members of the family.

Chromium

Available from the following companies:

Carlson®
Chelated Chromium
(Chelated Minerals)
Each tablet contains 200mcg of chromium provided from 9mg of chromium glycinate chelate and complex.

Carotec
Chromium Polynicotinate and Gymnema Sylvestre
Each capsule contains 150mcg of chromium polynicotinate and 300mg of gymnema sylvestre extract.

Source Naturals®
Chromium
Amino Acid Chelate
Each tablet contains 200mcg of chromium.

Chromium GTF
ChromeMate® Yeast Free
Each tablet contains 200mcg of chromium and 1.8mg of niacin

Ultra Chromium GTF™
Chromium Picolinate/ ChromeMate® Complex
Each tablet contains 100mcg of ChromeMate® chromium, 100mcg of chromium picolinate, and .9mg of niacin.

Tree of Life
Chromium Picolinate
Available in 200mcg and 400mcg tablets.

Coenzyme Q10

Available from the following companies:

Carlson®
Co-Q10
Available in 10mg, 30mg, 50mg,100mg and 200mg soft gels.

Carotec
CoQ-10
Each soft gel contains 100mg co-enzyme Q-10 with 50mg palm tocotirenols and 200mg of virgin coconut oil as the carrier.

Source Naturals®
Coenzyme Q10
Available in 30 mg and100 mg softgels.

Tishcon Corporation (raw goods supplier)
1-800-848-8442
www.tishcon.com/ *www.Q-Gel.com*

Hydrosoluble and high bioavailability. Comes in softsules® (soft gels).

Q-Gel®: 15 mg
Q-Gel® Forte: 30 mg
Q-Gel® Plus: with 50 mg alpha lipoic acid and 100 IU natural vitamin E
Q-Gel® Ultra: 60 mg
Carni-Q-Gel®: with 30 mg CoQ10 and 250 mg L-carnitine

Tishcon's CoQ10 products are available from the following companies:

Bio Energy Nutrients (a division of Whole Foods): 1-800-627-7775
Physiologics (a division of Whole Foods): 1-800-765-6775
CountryLife: 631-231-1031
Solanova: 1-800-200-0456
Phytotherapy: 201-891-1104
Nutrimedika: 1-800-688-7462
Swanson: 1-800-437-4148
Jordets: 1-888-816-7676
Epic: 1-800-848-8442
Optimum Health: 1-800-228-1507
Doctor's Preferred: 1-800-304-1708

Essential Fatty Acids

Omega Nutrition
Essential Balance
Omega's proprietary blend of five fresh-pressed oils, scientifically blended in the evolutionary 1:1 omega-3/omega-6 ratio. Contains certified organic flax, sunflower, sesame, pumpkin and borage oils. Also contains gamma-linolenic acid (GLA) and omega-6 fatty acids that diabetics often cannot produce. Available in liquid and capsules.

DHA (essential fatty acid)

DHA, an essential fatty acid necessary for life, is available in a non-fish, micro-algae form. Look for a product called Neuromins® DHA (in softgel form). Because of the importance of this product, several of the leading supplement companies are marketing Neuromins® DHA to retail stores. Listed below are companies—along with their customer service numbers—who can direct you where to obtain this product in your area:

BioDynamax (AMRION):	1-800-926-7525
Natrol®:	1-800-326-1520
Nature's Way:	1-800-962-8873
Solaray (Nutraceutical Corp.):	1-800-683-9640
Solgar:	1-800-645-2246
Source Naturals:	1-800-815-2333
Your Life (Leiner):	1-800-533-8482

Neuromins® DHA is available at healthfood stores everywhere, including the following:

Vitamin Shoppe:	1-800-223-1216
Vitamin World:	1-800-645-1030
Whole Food Markets:	1-800-901-0094
Wild Oats:	1-800-494-WILD

Mail-order sources for Neuromins® DHA:

Vitamin Shoppe:	1-800-223-1216
Puritan's Pride:	1-900-645-1030

On-line Sources for Neuromins® DHA (Search words: "Neuromins" or "DHA"):
www.vitaminshoppe.com
www.mothernature.com
www.drugstore.com
www.puritan.com

DHA Formulations for Children

Source Naturals®
Focus Child™
Chewable wafers, sweet and tart flavor. Contains 15mg DHA, 100mg magnesium, 2mg zinc, 310mg L-Aspartate, 100mg DMAE, and 50 mg standardized soybean lecithin.

Focus DHA™
Each kid cap™ (an easy-to-swallow soft gel) contains 100mg of
Neuromins® DHA.

Fish Oils (high in essential fatty acids)

Available from the following companies:

Carlson® Laboratories
Norwegian Cod Liver Oil
Bottled in liquid form. High in omega-3 and other essential fatty
acids and vitamin E. Available in natural and lemon-flavored.
Can be mixed into food.

Norwegian Salmon Oil
Each soft gel contains 1000 mg of salmon oil. Two softgels
provide 710 mg of total omega-3 fatty acids, including EPA (Eicosapentaenoic Acid), DHA (Docosahexaenoic Acid), DPA (Doco-
sapentaenoic Acid) and ALA (Alpha-Liolenic Acid).

Super-DHA™
Each soft gel contains 1000 mg of a special blend of fish body
oils, including menhaden and sardines, which are high in DHA
(Docosahexaenoic Acid) and EPA (Eicosapentaenoic Acid). This
product is unique because it supplies as much as 500mg of DHA
and 200mg of EPA.

Super Omega-3 Fish Oils
Contains a special concentrate of fish body oils from deep, coldwater fish, including mackerel and sardines, which are especially
rich in EPA and DHA. Each soft gel provides 570 mg of total
omega-3 fatty acids consisting of EPA (Eicosapentaenoic Acid),
DHA (Docosahexaenoic Acid), and ALA (Alpha-Liolenic Acid).

Prevail Corporation
1-800-248-0855
www.prevail.com
Eskimo-3®
Natural stable fish oil with vitamin E. Each serving of three soft
gels contains 500 mg of omega-3, 240 mg of EPA, 160 mg of
DHA, and 6.7 IU of vitamin E.

Flaxseed

Omega Nutrition
Hi-Lignan Nutri-Flax Capsules
Contains 550mg powder per capsule. A high-lignan fiber product with 7.9mg of lignans per three-capsule (1,650mg) serving. Lignans are the metabolism-balancing phytochemicals in flax. Flax seed fiber contains 30% more lignans than whole flax seed.

Green Tea Extract

Source Naturals®
Green Tea Extract
Each tablet contains 100 mg of standardized, patented Polyphenon 60™ green tea extract, providing at least 65 mg of polyphenols.

Gymnema Sylvestre

Available from the following companies:

Gaia Herbs, Inc.
1-800-831-7780
www.gaiaherbs.com
Gymnema Leaf, Ayurvedic (Gumar)
Concentrated liquid extract prepared from high quality gymnema leaf that is carefully shade-dried or naturally dry before the plant is picked.

Herbalists and Alchemists, Inc.
1-800-611-8231
Gymnema Sylvestre
Herbal extract available in various sizes.

Leukomeal (Muraglycine)

A highly concentrated extract obtained from lactobacilus bulgaricus that is a strong potentiator of insulin activity. Available in powder form. Contact Dr. Allan Sosin at 949-753-8889 or go to his website at *www.allansosinmd.com*.

Magnesium

Available from the following companies:

Carlson®
Magnesium
Each capsule contains 350mg of magnesium oxide.

Chelated Magnesium
(Chelated Minerals)
Two tablets contain 200mg magnesium provided from 1111mg magnesium glycinate chelate.

Liquid Magnesium
Each soft gel contains 400mg of liquid magnesium oxide.

Source Naturals®
Magnesium
Each tablet contains 825mg of malic acid and 152mg of magnesium.

Ultra Mag™
High Efficiency Magnesium Complex
Two tablets contain 400mg of magnesium and 50mg of vitamin B-6.

K-Mag C™
Each tablet contains 75mg of magnesium, 99mg of potassium, and 500mg of vitamin C.

Tree of Life
Magnesium
Available in 250mg tablets.

Mail Order

N.E.E.D.S.
1-800-634-1380
www.needs.com

N.E.E.D.S. carries a full line of quality supplements from top companies.

Multivitamin and Mineral Formulations for Children

Available from the following companies:

Body Wise®
Body Wise Tiger Vites™
Comprehensive vitamin and mineral supplement sweetened with natural fruit flavors—no sucrose and no artificial flavors or colorings. Chewable tablets with bubble gum flavor.

Carlson®
Scooter Rabbit
Chewable and tasty tablets containing 13 natural vitamins and 12 organic minerals. Sucrose-free.

Source Naturals®
Mega Kid™
A delicious chewable multivitamin for children ages 1-10. Contains a full complement of vitamins and minerals, and also includes Bioflavanoids, Bee Pollen, Papaya and Rutin. See bottle for correct dosage according to age.

Niacin

Available from the following companies:

Carlson®
Niacin
Available in 50mg, 100mg, and 500mg tablets.

Niacin-Time®
Each tablet provides a gradual release of 500mg over a period of 5 to 7 hours for sustained absorption that minimizes unpleasant side effects such as flushing or itching.

Tyler, Inc.
Niacinol™
One capsule provides 500 mg of niacin.

Niacinamide

Available from the following companies:

Carlson®
Niacin-Amide
Cellulose-coated tablets for ease of swallowing. Available in 100mg or 500mg.

Source Naturals®
Niacinamide
Available in 100mg and 1,500mg timed-release tablets.

Selenium

Enhances insulin activity by improving blood glucose control. Available from the following companies:

Carlson®
Selenium
Yeast-free. Each capsule contains organically bound selenium from L-selenomethionine, providing 200 mcg of selenium.

E-Sel
Natural-source vitamin E and organic selenium. Two soft gels contain 400 IU of vitamin E (d-alpha tocopheryl acetate derived from soybean oil) and 100 mcg of selenium (from L-selenomethione).

Source Naturals®
Selenomax®
Contains selenium from Selenomax® high selenium yeast. Available in 100 mcg and 200 mcg tablets.

Soy

Carlson®
Easy Soy Gold®
Each tablet contains 325mg of high soy isoflavone concentrate providing 130mg of soy isoflavones.

Vanadium

Available from the following companies:

Jarrow Formulas
Vanadyl Factors™
Each capsule contains 7.5mg of vanadium as vanadyl sulfate, 800mg taurine, and 100mg L-arginine.

N.E.E.D.S.
Vanadium
From Nutrisupplies
Pure vanadium in 250mcg tablets

Thorne
1-800-228-1966
www.thorne.com
Vanoxyl™
Contains vanadium as vanadyl sulfate. Available in 5mg and 25mg capsules

Vitamins A & D

Available from the following companies:

Carlson®
Vitamins A and D_3
Each soft gel contains 10,000 IU of natural source vitamin A and 400 IU of natural source vitamin D_3 from fish liver oil.

Source Naturals®
Vitamins A and D
Each tablet contains 10,000 IU of vitamin A and 400 IU of vitamin D.

Vitamin B Complex

Available from the following companies:

Carlson®
B-Compleet™
Provides all the B-vitamins plus vitamin C in a balanced formulation. Available in tablets.

Source Naturals®
Coenzymate™ B Complex
Contains coenzymes along with a full range of B-vitamins and CoQ10. Available in orange or peppermint flavored tablets that are taken sublingually (under the tongue) for direct absorption into the bloodstream.

Vitamin C

Available from the following companies:

Carlson®
Mild-C Chewable
Buffered form of chewable vitamin C that is non-acidic and gentle to the teeth. Each orange and tangerine flavored tablet supplies 250 mg of vitamin C and 28 mg of calcium.

MegaFood
Complex C
Vitamin C as found in food, is a very complex nutrient of which ascorbic acid is only one factor. Complex C DAILYFOODS® contains all the food factors, such as bioflavonoids, that occur in food and enhance its effectiveness. DAILYFOODS® FoodState® nutrients are 100% Whole FOOD and can be taken at any time throughout the day, even on an empty stomach. Available in 250 mg tablets.

Source Naturals®
C-500
Each tablet provides 500 mg of vitamin C (ascorbic acid) and 50 mg of rose hips.

C-1000 Timed Release
Provides a gradual release over a prolonged period of time. Each tablet provides 1,000 mg of vitamin C (ascorbic acid) and 100 mg of rose hips.

Wellness C-1000™
Each tablet contains 1,000 mg of vitamin C and several sources of bioflavonoids and alpha-lipoic acid.

Tree of Life®
Vitamin C with Rose Hips
Available in 500mg and 100mg tablets as well as 1,500mg timed-release tablets.

Ester-C with Bioflavonoids
Available in 500mg tablets

Vitamin C with Echinacea
Available in 500mg tablets

Vitamin C & Green Tea Extract
Each tablet contains 120mg of vitamin C and 100mg of green tea standardized extract. Also contains bioflavonoid complex.

Vitamin D

Available from the following companies:

Moss Nutrition
1-800-851-5444
Bio-D-Mulsion
An oil in water emulsion in which vitamin D has been dispersed. Each drop supplies 400 IU of emulsified vitamin D. If you wish to have your physician inquire about this product, they can call Moss Nutrition.

Carlson®
Vitamin D_3
Natural source vitamin D_3 from fish liver oil. Available in 400 IU and 1,000 IU soft gels.

Vitamin E

Available from the following companies:

Carlson®
E-Gems® Plus
Each soft gel contains vitamin E derived from soybean oil, supplying alpha-tocopherol plus substantial amounts of mixed tocopherols. Available in three strengths: 200 IU, 400 IU and 800 IU.

Carotec
Vitamin E
Each soft gel contains 200IU alpha tocopherol, 75mg gamma tocopherol, 28mg delta tocopherol, and 1mg beta tocopherol.

Tocomin®
Each soft gel contains 200mg of natural palm oil derived mixed tocotrienols.

Jarrow Formulas
Oil E
Vitamin E as 100% natural form d-alpha tocopherol with mixed tocopherols. Available in 400 IU and 600 IU soft gels.

MegaFood
E & Selenium DAILYFOODS®
In foods, vitamin E and selenium are always found together. Vitamin E doesn't work without the presence of selenium and vice versa. This combination offers these two important nutrients as they naturally occur in food, and therefore provides maximum protection. DAILYFOODS® FoodState® nutrients are 100% Whole FOOD and can be taken at any time throughout the day, even on an empty stomach. Each tablet contains 100 IU of vitamin E and 100 mg of selenium.

Source Naturals®
Vitamin E
Each softgel contains 400 IU of natural vitamin E (d-alpha tocopherol) and 67 mg of mixed tocopherols (d-beta, d-gamma, and d-delta). In a base of soybean oil.

Tree of Life®
Vitamin E (d-alpha form, natural)
Available in 400 IU and 1,000 IU soft gels.

Zinc

Available from the following companies:

Jarrow Formulas™
Zinc Balance 15
A synergistic combination of OptiZinc™ brand zinc monomethionate and copper gluconate in a 15mg:1mg zinc/copper ratio
because supplementing zinc without copper may cause copper
deficiency. Available in capsules.

Source Naturals®
OptiZinc®
Each tablet contains 30mg of zinc monomethionate and 300mcg
of copper sebacate.

Tree of Life®
Zinc
Available in 50mg tablets as well as zinc lozenges with echineacea
and vitamin C.

Special Resource Section (including foods, teas, juices, etc.)

Apple Sauce, Organic

Solana Gold Organics
1-800-459-1121
Organic pasteurized applesauce. Flavors: apple, gravenstein apple,
cinnamon crunch, as well as apple combined with other fruits
such as apricot, boysenberry, and others.

Beans

Beans are a rich source of protein, complex carbohydrates and soluble fiber, which has been scientifically proven to significantly lower blood sugar in Type 2 diabetics. Available from the following companies:

Internatural Foods, LLC
201-909-0808
Many Bean Soup
Contains a dozen different beans. Available in health and natural food stores.

Westbrae-Natural®
1-800-787-5090
Westbrae-Natural® has a wide variety of organic canned beans and organic bean soups, as well as Bearitos™ fat-free original baked beans, fat-free baked black beans, low-fat chilis, etc. Available in health and natural food stores.

Beef, Organic

Homestead Healthy Foods™
1-888-861-5670
www.homesteadhealthyfoods.com

Homestead Healthy Foods™ beef is raised in pastures on natural forages, which are certified organic and inspected annually by the certifier. Because it is raised on grass, the beef is high in omega-3 essential fatty acids. The meat is also lower in fat and free of any chemical residue, growth hormones, antibiotics or pesticides.

Bottled Water

Mountain Valley Water
1-800-643-1501
A fine, slightly alkaline water, bottled in glass from a pure, natural spring. Available in 5 gallon glass bottles and smaller sizes for easy-carrying.

Eggs

Gold Circle Farms™
1-888-599-4DHA
www.goldcirclefarms.com
Gold Circle Farms™ eggs are laid by hens that are fed a unique, all-natural, vegetarian diet—one that is enriched with DHA omega-3 and vitamin E. Two eggs provide 300mg of DHA—eight times more than ordinary eggs—as well as six times more of vitamin E and three times more of vitamin B-12.

Flaxseeds

Available from the following companies:

Health From The Sun
1-800-447-2229
FiPro FLAX™
Organic ground flaxseeds combined with fermented soy meal and other ingredients. Crunchy texture and delicious, nutty taste. Sprinkle on salads, cereal, soup and pasta. Available in healthfood stores.

Omega Nutrition
Flax Of Life—Cold Milled Organic Flax Seeds
Certified-organic flax seeds, vacuum-packed in a lined, resealable foil bag to retain freshness.

Flax Of Life—Whole Organic Flax Seeds
Certified-organic flax seeds.

Flourless Bread

Available from the following companies:

Food For Life
1-800-797-5090
Ezekiel Bread
Ezekiel Bread is produced from sprouted wheat and other grains, without a trace of flour. The sprouting process eliminates

the gluten from the wheat, so there is less chance of an allergic reaction. Best of all, the absence of flour gives the bread a lower glycemic index. Not only is it tasty, but you can safely make a sandwich using this highly nutritious bread without gaining weight or driving your blood sugar too high. Available in health food stores.

Internatural Foods, LLC
201-909-0808
Ryvita Crispbreads
Available in Tasty Light Rye and Tasty Dark Ryes. Contains no flour.

Goat Milk

Meyenberg® Goat Milk
1-800-343-1185
www.meyenberg.com
Meyenberg Ultra Pasteurized Fresh Goat Milk
Meyenberg Ultra Pasteurized Fresh Low-Fat Goat Milk
Meyenberg Aseptic (Tetra-Pak) Goat Milk
Meyenberg Powdered Goat Milk
Meyenberg Evaporated Goat Milk

Grains

Available from the following companies:

Bob's Red Mill
503-654-3215
www.bobsredmill.com
Millers, manufacturers and distributors of a wide range of grains and flour, including such exotic grains as amaranth and spelt.

Lundberg Family Farms
530-882-4550 (ext. 319)
www.lundberg.com
Grower and marketer of organic rice and rice products. They have an amazing variety of rices, rice cakes, etc. Reliable quality.

Green Drinks

Available from the following companies:

Greens +®
1-800-643-1210
www.greensplus.com

Greens +®
A whole living food containing concentrated sources of organic vitamins, minerals, essentials amino acids, phytochemicals, enzymes, co-enzymes, cell salts, chlorophyll, standardized herbal extracts, unique botanical extracts and soluble and insoluble plant fibers. Winner of the Peoples' Choice Award for the NNFA Market Place 2000.

Protein Greens+®
A synergistic blend of biologically complete protein isolates and the 29 nutrient-rich superfoods found in the award-winning Greens +®. Available in soy protein and whey protein formulas.

Tree of Life®
Advanced Greens
A blend of 29 nutrient-rich sea and land-based super-foods, herbs, fibrous ingredients and dairy-free probiotic cultures. Available in original and orange flavors. Naturally sweetened.

Advanced Greens with Protein
Contains soy and whey protein. Available in lemon-lime and cinnamon spice flavors.

Grinding Mill

Miracle Exclusives, Inc.
1-800-645-6360
www.miracleexclusives.com
Miracle Mill (Model ME821)
Stainless steel grinder for a wide variety of seeds and grains—including flax and soy beans. Convenient dial provides a range of adjustments from coarse to very fine grind.

Milk Products, Organic

Horizon
1-888-494-3020
Available in health food stores as well as many supermarkets.

Mixer

N.E.E.D.S.
Easy Mixer: battery operated mixer that effectively combines powders with liquids.

Noni

Tahiti Traders
1-800-842-5309
www.tahititraders.com
Tahiti Trader's Noni Juice
This juice acts as a tremendous aid for digestion and supports general health. Tahiti Trader's noni juice has an extremely high concentration of noni fruit per ounce.

Nuts and Seeds

Jaffe Bros.
760-749-1133
A large selection of organic nuts and seeds, as well as grains and beans.

Oatmeal

Internatural Foods, LLC
201-909-0808
McCann's Steel-Cut Irish Oatmeal
An excellent oatmeal that is nutritious and delicious. Available in boxes and tins.

Oils

Available from the following companies:

Omega Nutrition
Coconut Butter™
Contains 25% less fat than butter. Mild, light, creamy flavor makes this an excellent butter substitute.

Essential Balance Jr.
Omega's proprietary blend of five fresh-pressed oils, scientifically blended in the evolutionary 1:1 omega-3/omega-6 ratio. Contains certified organic flax, sunflower, sesame, pumpkin and borage oils. Also contains gamma-linolenic acid (GLA) and omega-6 fatty acids that diabetics often cannot produce. Formulated with a natural butterscotch flavoring that kids will love.

Flax Seed Oil
Unrefined and certified organic, grown without pesticides or artificial fertilizers and processed using Omega's exclusive omegaflo® process.

Olive Oil
Made from unrefined, extra-virgin olives that are fresh-pressed and omegaflo® bottled.

Tree of Life®
Tree of Life High Lignan Flax Oil
Contains all the antioxidants of their original Organic Flax Oil plus the added benefits of high fiber lignans. Bottled in liquid form. Available in health food stores.

Tree of Life Organic Extra Virgin Olive Oil

Bella Via Organic Extra Virgin Olive Oil
Made from the first pressing of 100% organic olives imported from the Andalusia region of Spain.

Pastas and Cake Mixes (Cake, Pancake, and Muffin)

Available from the following companies:

Omega Nutrition
Amaranth Pasta
From Mio Amore Pasta. Linguini from organic, gluten-free amaranth and organic flax meal.

Cake Mix—Chocolate and Vanilla
From Authentic Foods. All natural, gluten-free and super-moist. Includes brown rice flour, corn flour and bean flour (from garbanzo and broad beans).

Pancake and Muffin Mix
From Authentic Foods. A very versatile mix providing complete protein. Made from gluten-free bean flour and brown rice flour. Makes delicious pancakes, muffins and cookies.

Crum Creek Mills
1-888-607-3500
www.crumcreek.com
Crum Creek produces high protein pancake and muffin mixes, pastas and breadsticks, all made with added soy protein. Their products have less carbohydrates and more protein than similar products of their kind. They are a favorite of Dr. Sosin and his nutritionist because they have a low glycemic index and won't raise one's blood sugar. Crum Creek products can be purchased in health food stores.

Poultry

Sheltons Poultry, Inc.
1-800-541-1844
Free-range chicken and turkey with no added antibiotics. Available in natural foods stores.

Protein Bar

Ellis-Arnold Laboratories
1-888-357-8670
www.ealabs.com
Sugatrol RX™ (formerly Larabar)
This healthy food bar is used extensively by Dr. Sosin for his patients with diabetes and weight problems. Originally created by Diane Lara (the nutritionist who also created the recipes in this book) this special protein bar can be eaten by diabetics without raising their blood sugar. Dr. Sosin, Diane Lara and Dr. Michael Arnold have tested the bar repeatedly in diabetics and compared the blood sugar response with that from other protein bars. Only the Sugatrol RX™ bar had virtually no effect on blood sugar. Another clinical study was carried out under their direct supervision on Type 1 and Type 2 diabetics to determine the effect on blood sugar after ingesting Sugatrol RX™ , sugar-free candy and candy with sugar. The results showed conclusively that there was no appreciable rise in blood sugar levels in comparision to the sugar-free group or the sugar group.

Sugatrol RX™ is sweet, chewy and filling, and can be eaten as a snack without concern for blood sugar elevations. The secret is that its sweetness comes mainly from xylitol, a birch tree sugar that is slowly absorbed from the digestive tract and has a low glycemic index. Each bar contains an extensive blend of natural vitamins, minerals and digestive enzymes. It also contains almonds instead of peanuts and no milk.

Seafood

Available from the following companies:

Capilano Pacific
1-877-391-WILD (9453)
www.capilanopacific.com
Wildfish™
This company is a wonderful source for wild-caught salmon. Most of the salmon available in restaurants and stores are farm-

raised. Usually this means medications such as antibiotics have been added to the feed, as well as synthetic coloring. Wild-caught salmon has none of these problems and a high level of omega-3 fatty acids and much less fat than farm-raised salmon. It tastes better as well. Also available: halibut, tuna and lox without any added chemicals.

New World Marketing Group
203-221-8008
Sardines
Packed in pure virgin olive oil and virgin olive oil with garlic. Very high in omega-3 fatty acids. They also have water-packed sardines which contain less sodium. Available in natural foods stores.

Seafood Direct
1-800-255-5063
Salmon caught in the wild, including Wild Alaskan Salmon, King Salmon and Sockeye Salmon. Available in frozen filets and steaks. Also available in jars and cans.

Sea Salt

Omega Nutrition
Celtic Sea Salt
From the Grain & Salt Company. Harvested by a farmers' cooperative in Brittany, France, using a 2,000-year-old traditional Celtic method.

Stevia

Wisdom of the Ancients®
1-800-899-9908
www.wisdomherbs.com
Natural sweetener made from whole leaf Stevia (S*tevia rebaudiana Bertoni*) 6:1 concentrated extract. Available in concentrated tablets, liquid, and as a tea. Hundreds of scientific studies have been conducted on Stevia's effectiveness as a nutritional support for the pancreas.

Teas (Green)

Available from the following companies:

Great Eastern Sun
1-800-334-5809
www.great-eastern-sun.com
Haiku® Organic Japanese Teas

Organic Original Sencha Green Tea: the finest grade of green leaf tea available, made from the tender young leaves of selected tea bushes, cut at the peak of their flavor, rolled, steamed, and briefly dried. Contains 100% Nagata Japanese Organic Sencha Green Tea Leaves and Buds. Available in tea bags and bulk.

Organic Original Hojicha Roasted Green Tea: lower in caffeine than Sencha, Hojicha has a subtle smoky and rich flavor that is quite different from that of Sencha. Contains 100% Nagata Japanese Organic Hojicha Roasted Green Tea Leaves and Stems. Available in tea bags and bulk.

Triple Leaf Tea, Inc.
1-800-552-7448

Authentic traditional Chinese medicinal teas in tea bags, including different varieties of green tea. Triple Leaf has a wonderful natural method of decaffeinating green tea without using any chemical solvents. If you drink a lot of green tea and don't want caffeine, this is an ideal tea to use.

Tree of Life®

www.treeoflife.com
There are many fine healthfood stores all over the country that carry top-notch products. Many stores are supplied by an excellent company known as Tree of Life, a distributor of high quality natural foods at moderate prices. When shopping at healthfood stores, you can ask for Tree of Life products. If a store doesn't carry a particular product, they can order it for you.

Tree of Life Frozen Organic Vegetables
Certified organically grown.
Broccoli
Corn
Green Peas
Spinach

Tree of Life Frozen Fruit
Organic fruits are loaded with nutrients. These are often difficult
to obtain.
Strawberries
Blueberries
Raspberries

Tree of Life Frozen Smoothie Makers
Fresh-frozen chunks of 100% organic fruit. Ideal for juicing.
Banana, Rasberry, Strawberry

Tree of Life Organic Almond Butter
Available in two ways—creamy and crunchy—in glass jars.
Organic almonds are a good source of B-vitamins, vitamin E, essential fatty acids, calcium, and an array of other important minerals, as well as a substantial amount of protein.

Tree of Life Pasta Sauce
Original and Salt-Free—in glass jars.
This organic pasta sauce is made from vine-ripened, specially selected premium tomatoes that are grown for their sweetness and
flavor.

Tree of Life Organic Tamari and Shoyu
Made from organic soybeans and wheat. Excellent for steamed
vegetables and fish.
Shoyu
Wheat-Free Tamari

Harmony Farms Light Soymilk
Made from certified GMO-free soybeans. Available in orange or
vanilla flavors, enriched with extra vitamins and minerals.

Harmony Farms Soy Burgers
High in protein and isoflavones. Available in the following flavors: original, garlic, mushroom and onion.

McCann's Steel-Cut Irish Oatmeal
Available in boxes and tins.

Yogurt

The following two companies are sold by Oasis Sales and
Marketing. For more information on their products and where
to purchase them, call Oasis at 707-824-0119.

Brown Cow Yogurt
Yogurt is a good substitute for ice cream with only a third of the
fat and a third of the calories. It is also less allergenic than milk
because the lactose has been fermented. Brown Cow yogurt is
pasteurized but not homogenized and therefore safer for blood
vessels. It contains live active cultures and no steroids, bovine
growth hormone or antibiotics. Available in health food stores
and many supermarkets.

Redwood Hill Farm
707-823-8250
Goat Milk Yogurt
Made from pasteurized whole goat milk with live viable yogurt
cultures, Available in plain and different flavors, including vanilla,
apricot-mango, strawberry and blueberry.

Avoiding Environmental Toxins

In this book, you have learned importance of avoiding toxins in
the food you eat, the water you drink, the air you breathe, and in
virtually every product you use, from shampoos and toothpaste
to cleaning products for your home. The companies listed here

are of the highest quality. If you cannot find their products at your local health food store, please contact these companies directly for the store nearest you.

Dental Products

Woodstock Natural Products, Inc.
The Natural Dentist™
1-800-615-6895

Toothpaste: mint, cinnamon and fluoride-free mint
Mouth rinse: mint, cinnamon, cherry-flavored

According to Dr. Sosin, diabetics need to be especially vigilant about their teeth and gums because they have a tendency to develop periodontal disease. Woodstock Natural Products are formulated by a holistic dentist and contain soothing and healing herbs, with no alcohol, sugar, or harsh chemicals. These products have been clinically proven to kill germs that cause gum disease. In a study published in the *Journal of Clinical Dentistry* in 1998, researchers at the New York University College of Dentistry in New York City found that The Natural Dentist toothpaste removed plaque more effectively than the leading commercial brand. The same group also found that The Natural Dentist mouth rinse killed more germs than commercial brands.

Desert Essence®
1-888-476-8647
www.desertessence.com

Oral Care Collection
A complete line of antiseptic and cleansing oral care products using tea tree oil for deep cleaning and disinfecting of teeth and gums. All products are animal and eco-friendly and made without artificial colors, sweeteners or harsh abrasives.

Tea Tree Oil Dental Floss: creates a germ-free mouth and cleans between teeth

Tea Tree Oil Dental Tape: provides same benefits as floss with a wider ribbon
Tea Tree Oil Dental Pics: cleans between teeth with antiseptic power
Tea Tree Oil Breath Freshener: contains natural and organic essential oils

Removal of Mercury Amalgam Fillings

To find a holistic dentist who can safely remove mercury fillings, contact:

International Academy of Oral Medicine and Toxicology
Michael F. Ziff, D.D.S. Executive Director
P.O. Box 608531
Orlando, FL 32860
407-298-2450
(mercury-free dentists and physicians)

Jerome S. Mittelman, D.D.S.
263 West End Avenue, #2A
New York, NY 10023

Household Cleaning Products

Available from the following companies:

E Cover®
1-800-440-4925
Leading manufacturer of environmentally safe and toxic free household cleaning products. Their line includes dish and laundry products and a full range of household cleansers. Available in health food stores

Mail Order

N.E.E.D.S.
1-800-634-1380
www.needs.com
An excellent resource for top-notch environmental products, including the following:

Aireox Air Purifier (Model 45)
Removes mold spores, pollen dust, formaldehyde, and more.

Aireox Car Air Purifier (Model 22)
An unusual purifier for the car.

Allens Naturally
A full line of toxin-free household cleansers, including dishwashing and laundry detergents and all-purpose cleaners.

Water Filters
N.E.E.D.S. carries a variety of high-quality water filters

Elite Shower Filter and Massager
For removing chlorine, heavy metals and bacteria.

Natural Soaps

Available from the following companies:

Jason Natural Cosmetics
1-800-JASON-05
www.jason-natural.com

Jason Natural carries a full line of natural cosmetics that are free of toxic substances, including soaps, shampoos and underarm deodorants.
Chamomile Liquid Satin Soap™ with Pump
Natural Sea Kelp Shampoo
Aloe Vera Gel Shampoo

Omega Nutrition
Unscented Face and Body Soap
Made the old-fashioned way, in small batches using an early 1900's formulation. They Use only food grade oils, including unrefined omegaflo® oils.

Baby Shampoo
For sensitive skin and hair

Environmental Physician:

Dr. Sherry Rogers is a pre-eminent authority in environmental medicine who specializes in finding the environmental causative factors of disease. She is available for personal phone consultations (315-488-2856). One of her books, *Wellness Against All Odds*, is a must for all cancer patients. Get this and her other dozen books and referenced monthly subscription newsletter (free sample available) from 1-800-846-6687 or prestigepublishing. com.

Treatment for Diabetic Neuropathy

Vasomedical, Inc.
1-800-455-3327
www.eecp.com

EECP® MC2 Counterpulsation System

Dr. Sosin has used this device successfully for the treatment of diabetic neuropathy. This treatment is available at over 150 centers located in physicians' offices, clinics and hospitals throughout the United States.

Organizations that Recommend Integrative Care Practitioners

American Association of Naturopathic Practitioners
P.O. Box 20386
Seattle, WA 98112
703-610-9037

American College for Advancement in Medicine (ACAM)
P.O. Box 3427
Laguna Hills, CA 92654
1-800-532-3688

American Holistic Health Association
P.O. Box 17400
Anaheim, CA 92817-7400
714-779-6152
ahha@healthy.net

American Preventive Medicine Association
459 Walker Road
Great Falls, VA 22066
1-800-230-2762

Health Resource Newsletter
209 Katherine Drive
Conway, AR 72032
501-329-5272

National College of Naturopathic Medicine
11231 Southeast Market Street
Portland, OR 97216
503-499-4343

Society for Orthomolecular Medicine of America
2698 Pacific Avenue
San Francisco, CA 94115
415-346-2500

Glossary

Addiction—a physical and psychological dependence on a substance or behavior that is beyond voluntary control.

ADHD—Attention Deficit Hyperactivity Disorder. A disease entity attributed mainly to children who have difficulty focusing their attention on specific activities and cannot remain still.

Adrenal—a gland situated on top of the kidney. It produces the hormones cortisol, epinephrine, norepinephrine, DHEA, and small amounts of the sex hormones estrogen, progesterone, and testosterone.

Adult-onset diabetes—diabetes occurring in adults. The same as Type 2, insulin-resistant diabetes.

AGES (Advanced Glycation End Products)—products formed by the combination of body proteins with glucose. Glucose causes degeneration of these proteins so they do not function properly, and body tissues are damaged. The greatest damage occurs in the kidneys, the eyes, and the nerves.

Al dente—an Italian idiom indicating that a food has a firm consistency, often applied to pasta.

Alzheimer's disease—an increasingly common degenerative disease of the brain, leading to senility. The cause is unknown.

Amputation—removal of a part of the body, usually an arm or leg. In diabetes it occurs due to infection or severe circulatory compromise.

Antidepressants—medications used to treat depression. They often cause adverse reactions and may worsen depression.

Anti-nutrients—materials in food that offer no health benefits, but actually block the action of nutrients. Trans-fatty acids are anti-nutrients. So are lead, mercury, aluminum, pesticides, and herbicides.

Atherosclerosis—same as arteriosclerosis.

Arrhythmia—an abnormality of heart rhythm. Often benign, some forms are dangerous and require treatment.

Arteriosclerosis—occlusion of blood vessels by the progressive accumulation of fat and calcium, and active inflammation within blood-vessel walls.

Aspartame (Nutrasweet)—a calorie-free sweetener added to many foods, without nutrient value and with many potential side effects.

Autoimmune reaction—a situation where immune defenses are misdirected against the body's own cells, causing inflammation and illness.

Beta blockers—medications that lower blood pressure and reduce cardiac chest pain. They also interfere with blood-sugar control.

Biotin—a B vitamin important in glucose metabolism.

Blood sugar—glucose.

BMI (Body Mass Index)—a formula for assessing obesity. BMI = weight in kilograms divided by height (in meters) squared.

Calorie—the amount of energy, in the form of heat, required to raise the temperature of one gram of water by one degree centigrade. To lose a pound of fat you have to burn up 3,500 calories. An average teenager or adult consumes about 2,000 calories a day in food. So, if you eat nothing for two full days, you can lose about a pound in weight.

Cancer—uncontrolled growth of cells in the body. It is the result of both genetic and environmental factors. Thus, it can be significantly reduced. It is the second most common cause of death, next to heart disease.

Carbohydrates—compounds used as a source of energy. Also called sugars. Foods contain different forms of carbohydrates, such as lactose (milk sugar), fructose (fruit sugar), and maltose. These sugars can be converted by the body to form glucose, the primary fuel for cell metabolism. Sugar can be converted to fat, and vice-versa.

Carcinogenesis—the tendency to cause cancer.

Cardiac—referring to the heart.

Cardiovascular—referring to the heart and the blood vessels of the body.

Carotenoids—various forms of vitamin A.

Chelation therapy—an intravenous infusion of vitamins, minerals, and a chemical called EDTA, used in treating cardiovascular disease.

Cholesterol—a form of fat, produced only in the liver of animals, necessary for the production of sex hormones and cortisone, bile, and cell-membrane constituents. At high levels it contributes to atherosclerosis.

Chromium—a mineral normally present in the diet, which in larger amounts helps to increase the activity of insulin.

Claudication—pain occurring with exertion, usually in the legs, due to insufficient blood supply.

Coenzyme Q10—a chemical occurring in normal metabolism, especially important in heart muscle. Given as a supplement, it supports heart function and may have anti-cancer effects.

Coma—a state of unconsciousness from which one cannot easily be roused. It occurs due to metabolic disturbance, infection, or trauma.

Complex carbohydrates—simple carbohydrates combined with other materials, such as fiber, so that digestion and absorption are slower and blood-sugar elevations are more gradual.

Coronary—referring to the heart.

Cortisol—a hormone produced by the adrenal gland, released increasingly with stress, which helps to maintain blood sugar, blood pressure, and fluid and salt balance.

C-peptide—a protein by-product of insulin production, measured in the blood to assess insulin production. In Type 1 diabetes it is low. In Type 2 diabetes it is normal or high.

DHA (docosahexaenoic acid)—an omega-3 essential fatty acid, a major component of brain tissue.

DHEA (dehydropiandrosterone)—an adrenal hormone that supports brain, heart, and immune function, and serves as a precursor to other hormones.

Diabetes—an increasingly common disease in which the blood sugar is elevated due to lack of insulin production or, more commonly, resistance to the action of insulin.

Diuretics—medications that cause salt and water loss through the kidneys. They also raise blood sugar.

Enzyme—a protein that induces change in other substances. Digestive enzymes break down foods so they can be absorbed through the intestines.

EPA (eicosapentaenoic acid)—an omega-3 essential fatty acid.

Epinephrine—a hormone made by the adrenal gland, released during stress, which raises blood sugar, blood pressure, and heart rate, and increases alertness.

Fasting blood sugar—the level of blood sugar maintained in the fasting state, usually when a person has not eaten for at least five hours.

Fat—a greasy, soft material used by the body as a source of energy. Some forms of fat provide essential functions as components of body tissues.

Fiber—undigestible complex carbohydrates in plant foods that confer health benefits by regulating the rate of nutrient absorption and maintaining a favorable intestinal milieu.

Food additives—substances added to foods to enhance color or taste. The best known are MSG and aspartame. They may be toxic to humans.

Food preservatives—substances added to foods to keep them from spoiling. They may be toxic to humans.

Glucagon—a glucose-regulating hormone. Its action is counter to the action of insulin. It acts to stimulate glucose production by the liver when glucose levels fall too low.

Glucose—a form of sugar used by the body as its main energy source.

Glucose intolerance—a condition where blood sugar rises too high after eating carbohydrates. It is the same as insulin resistance. It often leads to diabetes.

GLUTS (glucose transporters)—specialized cellular components. When activated by insulin, they move from the inside of the cell to fuse with the cell membrane, allowing glucose to pass from the blood into the cell. GLUT is the door into the cell. Insulin is the key to the door.

Glycation—the combination of glucose with body proteins, resulting in interference with proper body functions. Higher blood sugars result in more glycation and more protein degradation.

Glycemic index—An important concept, indicating the rise in blood sugar caused by eating a particular food. The higher the glycemic index, the higher the blood sugar rises, and the more insulin is released to bring it back down again. Insulin is a fat-promoting hormone. Eating high-glycemic-index foods results in higher blood sugars, resistance to the action of insulin, and increasing obesity. Carbohydrate-rich foods, such as bread, have a high glycemic index, while foods high in protein and fat, such as beans, have a low glycemic index.

Glycohemoglobin—a compound formed by the combination of glucose with hemoglobin, a protein found in red blood cells. The level of glycohemoglobin reflects the average level of the blood sugar over the preceding 60 to 90 days. Thus, it provides information on how well diabetes has been managed in recent weeks.

Gout—painful swelling of joints due to deposition of uric acid, a breakdown product of certain proteins.

Grapeseed extract—a potent source of antioxidants.

Growth hormone—a hormone made by the pituitary gland in the brain that causes growth during childhood and adolescence. It also raises blood-glucose levels.

Gymnema sylvestre—an herb employed to increase insulin activity.

HDL (High Density Lipoprotein)—the component of cholesterol that prevents cardiovascular disease. "Good cholesterol."

Heart attack—death of cardiac tissue due to blockage of coronary blood vessels by arteriosclerosis.

Heavy metals—aluminum, lead, arsenic, mercury, and cadmium, found in various products and toxic to humans. May cause brain or kidney damage, or cancer.

Herbicides—poisons applied to crops to destroy unwanted vegetation. They are also toxic to humans. Organic products contain no herbicides.

HIV (Human Immunodeficiency Virus)—the cause of AIDS.

Heredity—characteristics passed on to an individual from its male and female parents, through the genes. Many medical conditions, such as Type 2 diabetes, have hereditary tendencies.

Hormone—a chemical messenger made in one organ that regulates the activities of other organs. For example, thyroid hormone controls the body's metabolic rate.

Hyperglycemia—high blood sugar.

Hypertension—high blood pressure. The increased pressure causes damage to the walls of blood vessels, leading to atherosclerosis, and to the heart, leading to heart failure.

Hypoglycemia—low blood sugar.

Hydrogenation—the chemical alteration of fats to make them solid at room temperature and keep them from becoming rancid. Hydrogenation creates dangerous by-products such as transfatty acids.

Hypercoagulable—tending to form blood clots easily. Heart attack and stroke are thus more likely to occur.

Insulin—A hormone, made in the pancreas, required for the entry of glucose into cells and the production of storage fat from glucose.

Insulin resistance—lack of adequate blood-sugar control by insulin. Thus, more insulin has to be made to keep the blood sugar down. Type 2 diabetes comes from insulin resistance. Relevant factors are obesity, inactivity, inadequate nutrition, and high-glycemic-index diets.

Islets of Langerhans—cells in the pancreas that make insulin.

Isoflavones—chemicals found in plants with beneficial effects in the human body. In particular they help to prevent cancer.

Juvenile-onset diabetes—diabetes in children. Once synonymous with Type 1, insulin-dependent diabetes. Now, however, juveniles also get Type 2, insulin-resistant diabetes.

Ketoacidosis—a complex metabolic imbalance, seen in poorly controlled Type 1 diabetes, when an acid state predominates. If not treated within a short period of time, it can be life threatening. It requires hospitalization for treatment with intravenous fluids and insulin.

Kidneys—organs that filter protein wastes and water from the body.

Leucotrienes—chemicals produced in the body that contribute to inflammatory and allergic reactions.

Lipoic acid (alpha lipoic acid, also called thioctic acid)—a component of normal metabolic pathways in the body. Given as a supplement it functions as an antioxidant, helps to control blood sugar, and protects the liver, eyes, and nerves.

LSD (Lysergic Acid Diethylamide)—a once-popular illicit drug, initially developed to treat psychiatric disorders. It causes visual aberrations and hallucinations, and may trigger insanity.

Master Settlement Agreement—an agreement reached between cigarette manufacturers and several states, involving payments of $206 billion in compensation for health damages caused by cigarettes.

Mellitus—sweet. Refers to the taste of urine in diabetes, which contains sugar.

Minerals—inorganic nutrients used by the body for various functions. The most important mineral are calcium, magnesium, sodium, potassium, and phosphorus.

MSG (monosodium glutamate)—a popular flavor enhancer with common adverse reactions including "Chinese Restaurant Syndrome."

Multiple sclerosis—an autoimmune neurologic disease characterized by weakness.

Muraglycine (Leukomeal)—a chemical derived from colonic bacteria that reduces inflammation. In diabetics it enhances insulin activity.

N-acetyl cysteine—a protein needed to produce glutathione, a compound essential for liver detoxification.

Neuropathy—disease affecting nerves, usually in the arms and legs, with resultant weakness, tingling, numbness, and pain.

Niacin—vitamin B_3.

Niacinamide—a form of niacin that may retard the development of juvenile diabetes if given early in the course of illness.

Nicotine—the chemical in cigarettes that causes addiction.

NIDDM—non-insulin-dependent diabetes mellitus. Diabetes due to resistance to the action of insulin.

Norepinephrine—a hormone made by the adrenal gland with very similar actions to epinephrine.

Nutrients—materials in food that support body structure and function. Proteins, fats, and carbohydrates are macronutrients, necessary in large amounts. Vitamins and minerals are micronutrients, necessary in small amounts.

Obesity—a condition of dangerous overweight. Having a Body Mass Index (kg./m^2) greater than 30.

Organic—relating to animals or plants. Also, containing the element carbon, required for all living things.

Organic foods—produced without using herbicides, pesticides, hormones, or antibiotics. Soils used to grow organic crops are richer in minerals than other soils, and the foods contain more nutrients.

Osmotic diuresis—increased production of urine by substances filtered through the kidneys that carry water with them. Glucose has this effect.

Osteoporosis—loss of calcium from bones, increasing the risk of fracture, especially of the hip, wrist, and lower spine.

Oxidation—a chemical reaction occurring during routine metabolic processes that may damage cells and cause illness.

Pancreas—a large organ located behind the stomach. It produces the hormones insulin, glucagon, and many digestive enzymes. In Type 1 diabetes, it is damaged so insulin is not produced. In Type 2 diabetes, it produces more insulin to compensate for resistance to the action of insulin.

Parkinson's disease—a degenerative brain disease with tremors, rigidity, and weakness.

PCP (phencyclidine)—a street drug that causes hallucinations and occasionally severe psychological disturbances and violent behavior.

Pesticides—poisons applied to crops to kill insects. They are also toxic to human beings. Organic products contain no pesticides.

Phosphatidylserine—an important component of nerve cell membranes. Often prescribed to enhance brain function.

Phytochemicals—chemicals found in plants. These chemicals may have beneficial (or toxic) effects on the people or animals that eat them.

Prostaglandins—physiologically active materials produced by various tissues with effects on blood vessel activity and muscle responsiveness in the lungs, uterus, and other organs.

Proteins—large molecules composed of amino acids, providing the major structural components of cells, also involved in immunologic function, muscle contraction, and enzyme activity. Proteins can be converted to carbohydrates or fats in order to produce energy, but they cannot be formed from fats or carbohydrates.

Psychiatric—referring to the treatment of mental disorders.

Psychoactive drug—one used to modify the state of consciousness or emotions.

Receptor—part of the cell membrane that binds with messenger molecules, so that activities within the cell are changed.

Renal—referring to the kidneys.

Retinopathy—disease affecting the retina, which is composed of layers of cells in the back of the eye that receive visual information and transmit it to the brain.

Salmonella—a bacterial organism often responsible for food poisoning, with symptoms of diarrhea, dehydration, and abdominal pain.

Seizure—a convulsion, occurring in diabetes when the blood sugar goes too low.

Serotonin—an important chemical mediator in the brain, derived from the essential amino acid tryptophan. Serotonin deficiency is considered a major cause of depression.

Simple carbohydrates—carbohydrates readily available for absorption, so that blood sugar rises quickly after eating.

Stress—reaction of the body to adverse forces, such as infection, injury, or death of a loved one. Stress adversely affects diabetic control and may precipitate illness.

Stroke—death of brain tissue due to loss of blood supply, leading to neurologic deficits such as paralysis or dementia.

Thorazine—a toxic psychiatric drug that once was the agent of choice for treating schizophrenia.

Thyroid—a gland in the neck that controls body metabolism through release of the hormone thyroxin.

Toxins—poisons. The higher up the food chain you go, the greater is the concentration of toxins. Animals retain toxins from the food they eat, in their fat cells. Meat from these animals may contain high concentrations of toxins.

Trace minerals—substances present in very small amounts, but nevertheless crucial for proper body functions.

Trans-fatty acids—an artificial type of fat created in food processing that increases cholesterol levels and promotes arteriosclerosis.

Triglycerides—a form of fat. They can be produced from sugar or transformed into sugar. High levels of triglycerides in the blood cause arteriosclerosis. They increase when the blood sugar is high, or when the diet contains simple sugars or alcohol.

Vanadyl sulfate—a mineral that enhances insulin activity.

Vascular—relating to blood vessels.

Vitamins—organic nutrients required by the body in small amounts for many different functions. They generally cannot be synthesized by the body, so must be supplied in the diet.

Water—a compound made of hydrogen and oxygen, which comprises 60 percent of total body weight. In uncontrolled diabetes, excessive water is carried out in the urine by the high concentration of sugar.

Selected References

Chapter 1—Getting the Facts Straight

Grady, Denise. New fronts in the war on diabetes in adults, *New York Times*, Sept. 7, 1999.

Grady, Denise. Too much of a good thing? Doctor challenges drug manual, *New York Times*, Oct. 10, 1999.

Grady, Denise. Doctors call for caution on 2 more diabetes drugs. Fears voiced at meeting on a banned drug, *New York Times*, May 20, 2000.

Guthrie, Diana W., and Guthrie, Richard A. *The Diabetes Sourcebook*, 3d ed., Los Angeles: Lowell House, 1997.

Komaroff (ed.), Anthony L. *The Harvard Medical School Family Health Guide*, New York: Simon & Schuster, 1999.

Koohestani, Niloofar et al. Insulin resistance and promotion of aberrant crypt foci in the colons of rats on a high-fat diet, *Nutrition and Cancer*, 29(1): 69-76, 1997.

Langreth, Robert, and Sharpe, Rochelle. Warner-Lambert drug avoids disaster before FDA panel but sales may suffer [Rezulin], *Wall Street Journal*, March 29, 1999.

Lazarus, J. et al., Incidence of adverse drug reactions in hospitalized patients, *JAMA*, 279(15):1200-1205, April 15, 1998.

Less risky treatment for diabetes is approved [Actos], *New York Times*, July 17, 1999.

Libov, Charlotte. *Beat Your Risk Factors*, New York: Plume, 1999.

Physician's Money Digest, October 1999 p. 33.

Rubin, Alan L. *Diabetes for Dummies*, Foster City, CA: IDG Books, 1999.

Saudek, Christopher D. et al., *The Johns Hopkins Guide to Diabetes for Today and Tomorrow*, Baltimore: Johns Hopkins, 1997.

Sharpe, Rochelle. Panel endorses diabetes drug by SmithKline [Avandia], *Wall Street Journal*, April 23, 1999.

Stolberg, Sheryl Gay. Stricter rules are urged on use of a diabetes drug [Rezulin], *New York Times*, March 27, 1999.

Thompson, Ginger. With obesity in children rising, more get adult type of diabetes, *New York Times*, Dec. 14, 1998.

Chapter 2—Diabetes Is a Family Affair

Daneman, Denis, Frank, Marcia, and Perlman, Kusiel. *When a Child Has Diabetes*, Buffalo, NY: Firefly, 1999.

McCool, Martha Hope, and Woodruff, Sandra. *My Doctor Says I Have a Little Diabetes*, Garden City Park, NY: Avery, 1998.

Nathanielsz, Peter W. *Life in the Womb: The Origin of Health and Disease*, Ithaca, NY: Promethean Press, 1999.

Singer, Alesia T. Barrett. *Coping with Your Child's Chronic Illness*, San Francisco: Robert D. Reed Publishers, 1999.

Touchette, Nancy. *The Diabetes Problem Solver*, Alexandria, VA: American Diabetes Association, 1999.

Chapter 3—The Great American Obesity Epidemic

Berger, Alisha. An early start for healthier habits, *New York Times*, July 20, 1999.

Davis, Mary C. et al. Hostile attitudes predict elevated vascular resistance during impersonal stress in men and women, *Psychosomatic Medicine*, 62:17, January/February 2000.

For youths, "vegetable" of choice is fried potato. *New York Times*, September 7, 1999.

Niaura, Raymond et al. Hostility and the metabolic syndrome in older males: the normative aging study, *Psychosomatic Medicine*, 62:7, January/February 2000.

Obesity rate rising fastest in the South, *New York Times*, Oct. 27, 1999.

Obesity studies from various researchers, *JAMA*, 282(16):1519-1588, Oct. 27, 1999.

Samaras, K. et al. Genetic and environmental influences on total-body and central abdominal fat: The effect of physical activity in female twins, *Annals of Internal Medicine,* 130(11):873-882, June 1999.

Chapter 4—High-Risk Foods

Ascherio, A. et al. Trans-fatty acids and coronary heart disease, *New England Journal of Medicine,* pp. 1994-1998, June 24, 1999.

Blaylock, Russell. *Excitotoxins: The Taste That Kills,* Santa Fe: Health Press, 1994.

Brody, Jane E. Increasingly, America's sweet tooth is tied to sour health, *New York Times,* Sept. 21, 1999.

Burros, Marian. Fears about fat prompt a call to improve the labeling on sugar, *New York Times,* Aug. 4, 1999.

Chase, Marilyn. Health journal: Amid new confusion, here's the truth about aspartame, *Wall Street Journal,* June 7, 1999.

Friedman, Milton. *Capitalism and Freedom,* Chicago: University of Chicago Press, 1962.

Georgieff, M. et al. Xylitol: An energy source for intravenous nutrition after trauma, *Journal of Parenteral and Enteral Nutrition,* pp. 199-209, 1985.

Hunt, Douglas. *No More Cravings,* New York: Warner Books, 1987.

Journal of Nutrition, pp. 1442-1449, Sept. 28, 1999.

Jump, Donald B. et al. Dietary fat, genes, and human health, in *Dietary Fat and Cancer,* edited by AICR, New York: Plenum, 1997.

Katan, Martijn B. Are there good and bad carbohydrates for HDL cholesterol?, *Lancet,* 353:1029-1030, March 27, 1999.

McCarthy, Laura Flynn. Much sweeter than sugar, but as safe?, *Rx Remedy,* pp. 10-11, July/August 1999.

O'Dea, Kerin, and Spargo, R.M. Metabolic adaptation to a low carbohydrate-high protein ("traditional") diet in Australian Aborigines, *Diabetologia,* 23:494-498, 1982.

O'Dea, Kerin. Marked improvement in carbohydrate and lipid metabolism in diabetic Australian Aborigines after temporary reversion to traditional lifestyle, *Diabetes,* 33:596-603, 1984.

Sahelian, Ray, and Gates, Donna. *The Stevia Cookbook,* Garden City Park, NY: Avery, 1999.

Whitaker, Julian. *The Memory Solution,* Garden City Park, NY: Avery, 1999.

Chapter 5—A Safer Environment

Casura, Lily Giambarba. Rx for winter health: Breathe green air, *Townsend Letter for Doctors & Patients,* pp. 68-74, December 1997.

Cohen, B.A., and Olsen, E.D. *Victorian Water Treatment Enters the 21st Century: Public Health Threats from Water Utilities' Ancient Treatment and Distribution Systems,* New York: Natural Resources Defense Council, 1994.

Kessel, Irene, and O'Connor, John T. *Getting the Lead Out: The Complete Resource on How to Prevent and Cope with Lead Poisoning,* New York: Plenum, 1997.

Lagnado, Lucette. Group sows seeds of revolt against genetically altered foods in U.S., *Wall Street Journal,* Oct. 12, 1999.

Laudan, Larry. *Danger Ahead: The Risks You Really Face on Life's Highway,* New York: Wiley, 1997.

Noble, Holcomb B. A debate over safety of softeners for plastic, *New York Times,* Sept. 28, 1999.

Pollack, Andrew. A disputed study suggests possible harm from genetically altered food, *New York Times,* Oct. 15, 1999.

Pusztai, Arpad, and Ewen, Stanley W.B. *Lancet,* Oct. 16, 1999.

Steingraber, Sandra. *Living Downstream: An Ecologist Looks at Cancer and the Environment.* Reading, Mass.: Addison-Wesley, 1997.

Strategic Plan for the Elimination of Childhood Lead Poisoning, Atlanta: Centers for Disease Control, 1991.

Unlabeled, untested . . . and you're eating it [Advertisement], *New York Times,* Oct. 18, 1999.

Upton, Arthur C., and Graber, Eden (eds.). *Staying Healthy in a Risky Environment: The New York University Medical Center Family Guide,* New York: Simon & Schuster, 1993.

Watering your body, *Rx Remedy,* pp. 18-23, July/August 1999.

Weil, Andrew. A healthier harvest, *Self Healing,* July 1998.

Wolverton, B.C. *How to Grow Fresh Air,* New York: Viking, 1996.

Chapter 6—Food as Medicine

American Diabetes Association & American Dietetic Association, *The New Family Cookbook for People with Diabetes,* New York: Simon & Schuster, 1999.

Behall, Kay M. et al. Effect of starch structure on glucose and insulin responses in adults, *American Journal of Clinical Nutrition,* 47:428-432, 1988.

Breslin, Margaret. A natural approach to diabetes, *Whole Foods,* May 1999.

Brody, Jane E. Vindication for the maligned fiber diet, *New York Times,* May 23, 2000.

Chandalia, Manisha et al. Beneficial effects of high dietary fiber intake in patients with Type 2 diabetes mellitus, *The New England Journal of Medicine,* 342 (19) May 11, 2000.

Edes, Thomas E., and Shah, Jayendra H. Glycemic index and insulin response to a liquid nutritional formula compared with a standard meal, *Journal of the American College of Nutrition,* 17(1):30-35, 1998.

Frost, G. et al. Glycaemic index as a determinant of serum HDL-cholesterol concentration, *Lancet,* 353: 1045-1048, March 27, 1999.

Hu, Frank B. et al. A prospective study of egg consumption and risk of cardiovascular disease in men and women, *JAMA,* 281(15):1387-1394, April 21, 1999.

Rendell, Marc. Dietary treatment of diabetes mellitus, *The New England Journal of Medicine,* 342 (19) May 11, 2000.

Romano, Rita. *Dining in the Raw,* New York: Kensington, 1992.

Salmeron, Jorge et al. Dietary fiber, glycemic load, and risk of non-insulin-dependent diabetes mellitus in women, *JAMA,* 277(6):472-477, Feb. 12, 1997.

Vital statistics, *Health,* p. 22, April 1999.

Wolever, Thomas M.S., and Jenkins, David J.A. The use of the glycemic index in predicting the blood glucose response to mixed meals, *American Journal of Clinical Nutrition,* 43: 167-172, January 1986.

Chapter 7—Exercise and Supplements

Anderson, Richard A. Effects of chromium on body composition and weight loss, *Nutrition Reviews,* 56(9):266-270, September 1998.

Boden, Guenther et al. Effects of vanadyl sulfate on carbohydrate and lipid metabolism in patients with non-insulin-dependent diabetes mellitus, *Metabolism*, 45(9): 1130-1135, 1996.

Brichard, Sonia M., and Henquin, Jean-Claude. The role of vanadium in the management of diabetes, *TiPS*, 16:265-269, 1995.

Ceriello, Antonio et al. Total plasma antioxidant capacity predicts thrombosis-prone status in NIDDM patients, *Diabetes Care*, 20(10):1589-1593, 1997.

Chausmer, Arthur B. Zinc, insulin and diabetes, *Journal of the American College of Nutrition*, 17(2):109-115, 1998.

Cunningham, John J. Micronutrients as nutriceutical interventions in diabetes mellitus, *Journal of the American College of Nutrition*, 17(1):7-10, 1998.

The evidence of omega-3s and heart disease, *Tufts University Health & Nutrition Letter*, p. 4, March 1997.

Fantus, George, and Tsiani, Evangelia. Multifunctional actions of vanadium compounds on insulin signaling pathways: Evidence for preferential enhancement of metabolic versus mitogenic effects, *Molecular and Cellular Biochemistry*, 182:109-119, 1998.

Fox, Gary N., and Sabovic, Zijad. Chromium picolinate supplementation for diabetes mellitus, *Journal of Family Practice*, 46(1):83-86, 1998.

Goodyear, Laurie J., and Kahn, Barbara B. Exercise, glucose transport, and insulin insensitivity, *Annu. Rev. Med.*, 49:235-261, 1998.

Halberstam, Meyer et al. Oral vanadyl sulfate improves insulin sensitivity in NIDDM but not in obese nondiabetic subjects, *Diabetes*, 45:659-666, May 1996.

Hayashi et al. Walking to work and the risk for hypertension in men: The Osaka Health Survey, *Annals of Internal Medicine*, 130:21-26, 1999.

Isbir, T. et al. Zinc, copper and magnesium status in insulin-dependent diabetes, *Diabetes Research*, 26:41-45, 1994.

Jacob, S. et al. Enhancement of glucose disposal in patients with Type 2 diabetes by alpha-lipoic acid, *Arzneim.-Forsch./Drug Res.*, 45(II)(8):872-874, 1995.

Jacob, Stephan et al. The antioxidant alpha-lipoic acid enhances insulin-stimulated glucose metabolism in insulin-resistant rat skeletal muscle, *Diabetes*, 45:1024-1029, 1996.

Jakicic, John M. et al. Effects of intermittent exercise and use of home exercise equipment on adherence, weight loss, and fitness in overweight women, *JAMA*, 282(16):1554-1560, Oct. 27, 1999.

Kao, W.H. Linda et al. Serum dietary magnesium and the risk for Type 2 diabetes mellitus: the artherosclerosis risk in communities study, *Archives in Internal Medicine*, 159(18): 2151-2159, October 11, 1999.

Lancet, 350 (9071):81, July 12, 1997.

Mertz, Walter. Interaction of chromium with insulin: A progress report, *Nutrition Reviews*, 56(6):174-177, 1998.

Nader, Philip R. et al. Three-year maintenance of improved diet and physical activity: the CATCH Cohort, *Archives of Pediatric and Adolescent Medicine*, 153(7), July 1999.

Packer, Lester, and Coleman, Carol. *The Antioxidant Miracle*, New York: Wiley, 1999.

Sosin, Allan, and Jacobs, Beth Ley. *Alpha Lipoic Acid*, New York: Kensington, 1998.

Verma, Subodh et al. Nutritional factors that can favorably influence the glucose/insulin system: Vanadium, *Journal of the American College of Nutrition*, 17(1):11-18, 1998.

von Schacky, Clemens et al.The effect of dietary omega-3 fatty acids on coronary atherosclerosis, *Annals of Internal. Medicine*, 130:554-562, 1999.

Vuksan,Vladimir et al. American ginseng (panax quinquefolius L) reduces postprandial glycemia in nondiabetic subjects with Type 2 diabetes mellitus, *Archives of Internal Medicine*, 160(7), April 10, 2000.

Wallace, Edward C. Diabetic epidemic, *Energy Times*, pp. 24-28, April 1999.

Wei, Ming et al. The association between cardiorespiratory fitness and impaired fasting glucose and Type 2 diabetes mellitus in men, *Annals of Internal Medicine*, 130(2) 89-95, Jan. 19, 1999.

Wei, Ming et al. Low cardiorespiratory fitness and physical inactivity as predictors of mortality in men with Type 2 diabetes, *Annals of Internal Medicine*, 132(8) 605-611, April 18, 2000.

Chapter 8—Parents and Children: Partners In Healing

The Diabetics Control and Complications Trial Research Group. The effect of intensive treatment of diabetes on the development and progression of long-term complications in insulin-dependent diabetes mellitus, *New England Journal of Medicine*. 1993; 329:977-986.

UK Prospective Diabetes Study Group. Intensive blood-glucose control with sulphonylureas or insulin compared with conventional treatment and risk of complications in patients with Type 2 diabetes (UKPDS 33), *Lancet* 1998; 352: 837-853.

For Further Reading

Bernstein, Richard K., M.D. *Dr. Bernstein's Diabetes Solution: A Complete Guide to Achieving Normal Blood Sugars*. Boston: Little Brown and Company, 2000.

Broadhurst, C. Leigh, Ph.D. *Diabetes: Prevention and Cure*. New York: Kensington, 1999.

Galland, Leo. *Superimmunity for Kids*. New York: Delacorte, 1989.

Meyerowitz, Steve. *Power Juices, Super Drinks*. New York: Kensington, 2000.

Pescatore, Fred, M.D. *Feed Your Kids Well: How to Help Your Child Lose Weight and Get Healthy*. New York: John Wiley and Sons, 2000.

Pitchford, Paul. *Healing With Whole Foods*. Berkeley: North Atlantic Books, 1996.

Romano, Rita. *Dining in the Raw: Ground-Breaking Natural Cuisine That Combines the Techniques of Macrobiotic, Vegan, Allergy-Free, and Raw Food Disciplines*. New York: Kensington, 1997.

Index

acidosis, 24, 29–30, 33
Actos, 32
adrenal insufficiency, 12
adult-onset (type-2) diabetes, 4, 6,
    10, 15, 18–19
    benefits from tight control of,
        144
    blood sugar levels and, 70
    in children, 19–21
    complications from, 27
    diagnosing, 21
    drug approach for, 29–30
    fiber and, 107–8
    first symptoms of, 21–22
    genetics in, 22
    heredity and, 12
    individuals at high risk for devel-
        oping, 22
    insulin for, 14
    link between hostility, fat, and,
        51–52
    obesity and, 18, 67, 120, 122
    outlook for, 28
    pharmaceutical approach to
        treating, 147
    physical activity, 119, 124
    Pima Indians and, 53
    type-2, non-insulin-dependent
        diabetes, 19
advanced glycosylation end prod-
    ucts (AGES), 25
alpha lipoic acid, 132–33
alpha-glucosidase inhibitors, 30

American Diabetes Association, 124
amylase, 151
Annals of Internal Medicine, 119, 120
antibiotics, 90–91
antioxidants, 129–33
arachidic fatty acids, 64
Archives of Family Medicine, 157
Archives of Internal Medicine, 136
Archives of Pediatric and Adolescent
    Medicine, 125
arteriosclerosis, 51, 65
artificial sweeteners, 76–77
Ascherio, A., 66
aspartame, 76–77
aspartic acid, 76
atherosclerosis, 16, 17, 27, 59
athletes, diabetic, 124
autoimmune diseases, juvenile dia-
    betes and other, 12
Avandia, 32

B vitamins, 136
Bates, David, 34
benzoic acid derivatives, 30
beta cells, 9, 11
biguanides, 29–30
Billie Jean King Foundation, 124
biotin, 136
blindness, 23
blood sugar levels, 7
    diet and blood-sugar
        fluctuations, 105–6
    ginseng and, 136–37

blood sugar levels (*cont.*)
    high blood sugar, 8–9
    low blood sugar, 8, 9, 23–24
    processed carbohydrates and, 70
body fat, 119–20
body mass index (BMI), 47, 48–49, 50

C-peptide, 12, 21
calcium, 62, 63
    alternative sources of, 99
calcium channel blockers, 32
cancer
    cow's milk and ovarian, 63
    obesity and, 50, 57–58
carbohydrates and sugar, processed, 69–70
cardiovascular disease
    cardiac and cerebrovascular disease, 26–27
    dietary programs for heart disease, 64
    preventing, 17–18
cataracts, 63
cellulose, 70
Centers for Disease Control (CDC), 47
challenge of diabetes, 34–35
chelation, 26
Chinese restaurant syndrome, 80
cholesterol
    cardiovascular disease and, 17
    child's cholesterol level, 65
    HDL, 64, 100, 108
    levels among Americans, 82
chromium, 134–35
claudication, 25
coenzyme Q10 (CoQ10), 131–32
Cohen, Jay S., 34
complex carbohydrates, 69–70
Consumer Reports, 89
cortisol, 8

d-alpha tocopherol, 130, 131
daidzein, 58
Diabetes, 22
diabetes management, your child and, 41–42
    demystifying diabetes management, 43–45

diabetes mellitus, 10
diabetic ketoacidosis, 21, 24
diet and blood-sugar fluctuations, 105–6
dietary fats, 64–65
diketopiperazine (DKP), 77
docosahexaenoic acid (DHA), 100, 137
Donnelly Awards, 124
drugs
    drug approach for type-1 and type-2 diabetes, 28–30
    drug dangers, 30–32
    pharmaceutical advances in controlling diabetes, 146–47
    the right approach to, 34
    side effects from diabetic, 30–31, 33

eggs, 99–101
eicosapentaenoic acid (EPA), 137
enhanced external counterpulsation (EECP), 26
enriched flour, 71
Enrichment Act of 1942, 71, 166
environmental issues
    environmental toxins, 90–91
    genetically engineered foods, 88–89
    pesticides, 87
    water, 83–87
epinephrine, 8
essential fatty acids, 64, 137–38
estrogen, 51
exchange lists, 106
excitotoxins, 77
exercise and supplements
    antioxidants, 129–33
    B vitamins, 136
    essential fatty acids, 137–38
    exercise and insulin, 123–24
    get your family moving, 122–23
    getting into the exercise habit early, 125
    gymnema sylvestre, 136
    hypoglycemia and exercise, 23
    importance of exercise over diet, 119–20
    incorporating exercise, 148–49
    Justin's story, 138–40

Kara's story, 4, 120–21
minerals, 133–36
promote daily sports and exercise, 158
role of supplements, 126–27
special nutrients for diabetic children, 127–29
sports, 125
eye complications and eye diseases, 143–44

faces of diabetes, 3–6
family dynamics, 36
changing the family dynamic, 40–41
considering home schooling, 42–43
demystifying diabetes management, 43–45
gaining control, 38
how fear paralyzes learning, 38–40
involving your child in diabetes management, 41–42
questions and answers on childhood diabetes, 36–37
fasting, blood-sugar levels and, 8
fasting state, 6
fat hormone, exercise and, 122
Feeding Your Child for Lifelong Health (Roberts and Heyman), 62
fiber
to control blood sugar, 106–7
glycemic index and high-fiber foods, 108
high-fiber diets, 68
plant, 70–71
filters, water, 86
food
breakfast recipes, 167–74
containing fiber, 106–7
dessert recipes, 186–93
dinner recipes, 177–86
drinks, 195
eat at home, 157
encouraging proper chewing, 151
ensuring a proper diet, 152–53
fast food, 54–57, 64, 66
food labels, 74, 165–67

genetically engineered foods, 88–89
have meals together, 157–58
helpful nutritional hints, 162–67
helping kids make wise food choices, 147–48
high-glycemic-index foods, 5, 23, 101, 106
insulin and weight gain, 50
low-glycemic-index foods, 101, 106, 111
lunch recipes, 174–77
natural foods, 57
organic foods, 88, 91
potatoes, 58–60
principles of good nutrition, 153–54
proper eating/shopping guide, 197–200
snacks, 193–95
soy products, 58
food additives, 90
Food and Drug Administration (FDA), U.S., 31–32, 73, 77, 165
food enhancers, 79–81
food as medicine, 95
alternative sources of calcium, 99
anti-diabetes diet, 102–3
diet and blood-sugar fluctuations, 105–6
eggs, 99–101
exchange lists, 106
fiber, 106–8
glycemic index, 108–13
good foods/bad foods, 97–99
managing diabetes, 117–18
overcoming dietary misinformation, 114–17
putting it all together, 103–4
taking the initiative, 101–2
weight control, 96–99
Wendy's story, 104–5
Zach's story, 101–2
Food and Nutrition Board, 126
foods, high risk
artificial sweeteners, 76–77
aspartame, 76–77
the business of food, 81–82
dietary fats and diabetes, 64–65

foods, high risk (*cont.*)
  enriched flour, 71
  food enhancers, 79–81
  high-fat diet, 63–64
  high-protein diet problems,
    67–69
  milk, 61–63
  MSG, 80–81
  processed carbohydrates and
    sugar, 69–70
  stevia, 78–79
  sugar, 71–76
  sweet solutions, 78–79
  trans-fatty acids, 65–67
  whole grains and vegetables,
    70–71
  xylitol, 77–78
formaldehyde, 77
formic acid, 77
Friedman, Milton, 81

Genetic ID, 89
genetically engineered foods, 88–89
genetically modified organisms
  (GMOs), 88
genetics
  role of, 22–23
  weight gain and, 52–53
genistein, 58
Georgieff, M., 78
ginseng, 136–37
glucagon, 8, 24
Glucophage, 33
glucose, 6, 7, 8, 10
glucose tablets, 123
glucose tolerance factor (GTF), 135
glucuronidase, 57–58
Glutamate, 80
glycation, 132–33
glycemic index, 108, 111–12
  of common foods, 109–10
  high-glycemic-index foods, 5, 23,
    101, 106, 111–12, 113
  low-glycemic-index foods, 101,
    106, 111
  making the index work for you,
    112–13
  using the, 108, 111
glycitein, 58
glycogen, 7, 8

goat's milk, 63
Goland, Robin S., 20
growth hormone, 8
gymnema sylvestre, 136

Heyman, Melvin, 62
high blood pressure, 17, 25
high-fiber diets, 68
high-glycemic-index foods, 5, 23,
  101, 106, 111–12
high-protein diet problems, 67–69
home schooling, 42–43
homocysteine, 17
hormone replacement therapy, 51
hospitals, food served in, 56
hydrogenation, 65
hyperbaric oxygen, 26
hypoglycemia, 23–24
  exercise and, 23, 123
  reactive, 10, 23
  risk of tight diabetic control and,
    144
  as side effect of sulfonylureas, 29,
    31
hypoglycemic reactions, 5
hypothyroidism, 12

insoluble fiber, 70
insulin, 3, 5, 14–15, 30
  blood sugar levels and insulin
    insensitivity, 70
  C-peptide and, 12
  enhancers and blockers, 11
  exercise and, 123–24
  given intranasally, 146
  honeymoon period, 15, 129
  insulin dependence and adopt-
    ing a lifestyle program,
    15–16
  and weight gain, 50–51
  what insulin does, 9–10
isoflavones, 58

Jones, Kenneth L., 20
*Journal of the American Medical
  Association*, 54, 69
juvenile (type-1) diabetes, 3, 5, 6,
  10, 15, 18, 83, 141
  complications from, 27
  cow's milk and, 62

diagnosing, 13
drug approach for, 28–29
heredity and, 12
outlook for, 16
physical activity, 119, 124
possible triggers of, 11–12
tennis awards, 124
type-1, insulin-dependent diabetes, 19

ketoacidosis, 21, 24
ketones, 5, 24
ketosis, 67–68
kidneys, kidney functions and
  blood-sugar levels, 8, 144

lactic acidosis, 29–30, 33
lactose, 61, 62
Lancet, The, 89
Lara, Diane, 162
lecithin, 100
leptin, 122
Levins, Gloria Olivas, 125
lignins, 58, 70
lipoic acid, 132–33
lispro, 14
long-term complications, preventing, 23–27
low blood pressure, 25
low-glycemic-index foods, 101, 106,
  111
lymphocytes, 11

magnesium, 53, 133–34
margarine, 65–66, 81–82
metformin, 29
methanol, 76–77
microvasculature, 26
milk, 61–63
minerals, 133–36
Misbin, Robert, 32
misinformation, dietary, 114–17
  ignore false information, 154–55
monosodium glutamate (MSG),
  80–81
Mothers Against Drunk Driving
  (MADD), 159
muraglycine, 101–2
myasthenia gravis, 12
myristic saturated fatty acids, 64

Nader, Philip R., 125
National Heart, Lung, and Blood
  Institute, 46–47, 125
National Institutes of Health, 32
National Soft Drink Association, 73
National Task Force on the
  Prevention and Treatment of
  Obesity, 50
Nestle, Marion, 73
neurologic impairment, 23
neuropathy, 21, 87
New England Journal of Medicine, 107
Niaura, Raymond, 51–52
nicotinamide, 14
non-insulin-dependent diabetes
  mellitus (NIDDM), 18
non-resistant starches, 69–70
norepinephrine, 8
Nutrasweet, 76–77
nutritional program, 162
  breakfast recipes, 167–74
  dessert recipes, 186–93
  dinner recipes, 177–86
  drinks, 195
  helpful hints, 162–67
  lunch recipes, 174–77
  snacks, 193–95

obesity, 46
  blood sugar levels and, 70
  and cancer, 57–58
  diet and, 67
  energy equation, 53
  fast food, 54–57
  genetics, 52–53
  insulin and weight gain, 50–51
  measuring, 46–50
  other factors, 51
  television and, 54
  type-2 diabetes and, 18, 67, 120,
    122
omega-3 fatty acids, 64, 65, 137, 138
omega-6 fatty acids, 65, 137–38
organ damage, 24–25
organic foods, 88
osmotic diuresis, 8, 84
osteoporosis, 62

pancreas, 6, 9–10, 18
  pancreatic cells, 12

pancreas (*cont.*)
  pancreatic damage and the onset
    of diabetes, 13–14
  transplants, 146
  of type-2 diabetics, 20
parents and children
  Brian's story, 141–45
  a child's health crisis can draw
    the family closer, 150–51
  developing good health habits,
    151–52
  encouraging children to share
    their feelings, 149–50
  helping kids make wise food
    choices, 147–48
  incorporating exercise, 148–49
  Jackie's story, 160–61
  parents' questions about getting
    well, 145–46
  pharmaceutical advances in con-
    trolling diabetes, 146–47
  reinforcing healthy decisions,
    149
  28 tips for keeping your child
    healthy, 152–60
  using nutritional supplements,
    148
partially hydrogenated vegetable
  oils, 65
pectins, 70
peripheral vascular disease, 25–26
pernicious anemia, 12
pesticides, 87
pharmaceutical advances in controlling diabetes, 146–47
phenformin, 33
phenylalanine, 76
Physicians' Desk Reference (PDR), 30,
  34
Pima Indians, genetic defect in, 53
polyunsaturated fatty acids, 65
Postgraduate Medicine, 34
protein, high-protein diet
  problems, 67–69
Psychosomatic Medicine, 51
pyridoxine, 136

questions and answers on
  childhood diabetes, 36–37,
    145–46

reactive hypoglycemia, 10, 23
recommended daily allowance
  (RDA), 126
"Reducing Children's Television
  Viewing to Prevent Obesity: A
  Randomized Controlled Trial"
  (study), 54
Rendell, Marc, 107–8
resistant starches, 69
retinopathy, 24
Rezulin, 30, 32–33
rice milk, 63
Robert, Susan, 62
Robinson, Thomas N., 54

Salmeron, Jorge, 69
sleep deprivation, 151–52
smoking, 90
  weight gain and, 51
soft drinks, 56, 165
soluble fiber, 70
soy milk, 63
soy products, 58
starches, 69–70
stearic fatty acids, 64
stevia, 78–79
stress
  blood-sugar levels and, 8, 13–
    14
  weight gain and, 51
stress hormones, 8
strokes, 26–27
sudden infant death, 62
sugar
  America's consumption of, 72
  and empty calories, 71–72
  identifying hidden sugars on
    food labels, 74
  processed carbohydrates and,
    69–70
  sugar facts, 74–75
  sugars added to foods, 73
  turning kids into sugar junkies,
    75–76
sulfonylureas (SUs), 29, 31
super eggs, 100
supplements
  exercise and role of, 126–27
  give your child vitamin and min-
    eral supplements, 156–57

special nutrients for diabetic
    children, 127–29
using nutritional, 148
surgical therapy, 26
Syndrome X, 4, 120

television
    commercials for fast-food, 56
    and obesity, 54
tennis awards, 124
thiamin, 136
thiazolidinediones, 30
thyroiditis, 12
toxins, environmental, 90–91
trans-fatty acids, 64, 65–67, 82
triglycerides, 7, 17, 64, 65, 108
type-1 diabetes. *See* juvenile (type-1)
    diabetes
type-2 diabetes. *See* adult-onset
    (type-2) diabetes

vanadium, 135–36
vascular diseases, 64–65
vegetables and whole grains, 70–71
viral infections in children, 141
visual loss, 21–22
vitamin C, 8, 130
vitamin D, 14

vitamin E, 130–31
vitamins
    for early prevention, 14
    water-soluble, 8
vitamins, B, 8, 14, 136
vitiligo, 12
Vuksan, Vladimir, 136–37

Wall Street Journal, 88
water
    how pure is your drinking?,
        85–86
    lifelong need for, 84–85
    as the preferred beverage, 112
    promotes weight loss, 85
    purifying your drinking, 86
    tap, 87
    your drinking, 83–84
Wei, Ming, 120
weight control and diabetes man-
    agement, 96–99
Weil, Andrew, 88
what is diabetes?, 6
whole grains and vegetables, 70–71
World Health Organization, 85

xylitol, 77–78

About the Authors

Allan Sosin, M.D., graduated from Northwestern University Medical School. He is board certified in Internal Medicine and Nephrology. From 1982 to 1995, he established a private practice in Philadelphia, during which time he became increasingly involved in nutritional and alternative therapies. Also during this time, Dr. Sosin served as assistant medical director for the Institutes for the Achievement of Human Potential in Philadelphia, where he treated brain-injured children for 14 years. In 1995, he and his family moved to California, where he became medical director of the Whitaker Wellness Institute in Newport Beach. He now works at the medical center he founded in Irvine, California, which integrates traditional with alternative approaches.

Dr. Sosin can be reached at:
Sand Canyon Medical Center
16100 Sand Canyon Avenue, Suite 240
Irvine, CA 92618
Phone: 949-753-8889
Fax: 949-753-0410
www.allansosinmd.com

Sheila Sobell is an award-winning health writer. She is the author of *The Smart Guide to Sports Medicine* and co-author of *Slim & Fit Kids: Raising Healthy Children in a Fast Food World.* She is based in Atascadero, CA at *www.writersobell.com.*